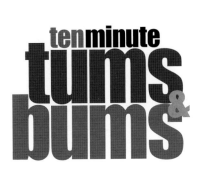

ten minute tums & bums

GLORIA THOMAS

CASSELL&CO

For my sisters
Carol Marie Stone and Bridgette Grace Bridge

First published in the United Kingdom in 2001 by Cassell & Co

All photography by Bill Morton, apart from page 17: both copyright
© Science Photo Library

A CIP catalogue record for this book is available from the British Library

ISBN 0 304 35477 5

Art Editor: Austin Taylor
Designer: Helen James

Printed and bound in Italy by Printer Trento S.r.l.

Cassell & Co
Wellington House
125 Strand
London WC2R 0BB

NOTE
If you have a medical condition that could be adversely affected by exercise,
check with your doctor before embarking on any exercise programme.

contents

introduction

During all my years working in the exercise industry, no other area of the female body has ever attracted as much attention as the **problematic bum and tum**. Studio timetables are littered with 'BT' – no, nothing to do with a national telephone company, but specialist classes that focus on targeting those areas of the body with which most women seem to have a **never-ending fascination**, their bum and tum.

Clients would come in their droves to these bum and tum classes, more so than to any other.

I wondered – perhaps rather cynically – if they were trying to avoid getting hot and sweaty in aerobics classes or working on those horrid-looking machines in the gym.

But, after spending many hours **discussing, gossiping and observing** women poking, prodding and scrutinising themselves in the cloakroom mirror, I have come to the conclusion that the bum and tum are the areas on a woman's body that are the most **sensual and desirable** at their best, and the most unattractive and unsightly at their worst.

In our view of the world, lean, toned, shapely bums and tums make us look younger, stronger and sexier.

I first became aware of the condition of my tum and bum following the birth of my son. During the first half of my pregnancy I had happily eaten my way through stacks of cheese-and-pickle sandwiches, king-size burgers and coffee milkshakes. I then spent most of the second half on my back with complications which resulted in a premature delivery. During that time I ate everything in sight, from the hospital food to the daily takeaways that were brought in to appease me while I was waiting to deliver. The result was that by the time my son was born I had put on 19 kg (3 stones). I was overweight and very prone to baby blues.

Breastfeeding helped my tummy muscles knit back together and eradicate a few of the dimples around my bum, but then I discovered exercise and good nutrition. The weight went fairly quickly and I started to feel better within myself – so much so that I decided to become an exercise teacher. Over the years I have managed to keep my tum and bum in pretty good shape through my work – but now, 13 years later, I am teaching less and spending more time writing and exploring different concepts for health and fitness. My life has started to become sedentary once again, with the result that, horror of horrors, rolls of flesh are beginning to accumulate around my middle. I find myself poking and prodding and leaning forwards and sideways, exploring those intriguing folds and dimples on my lower half.

My son laughingly suggests that I am getting old. He may have a point: I am getting *older*. And I must confess that his comment prompted me to spend a thoughtful hour or two considering the process of ageing. I have come to the conclusion, however, that the rolls of flesh that are just beginning to make themselves at home around my tum have less to do with age and more with my lifestyle. Having reduced my physical workload, I am no longer as active as I was, and I spend more time at my laptop computer. That, and the fact that I am the eternal student, taking one course after another, means I am sitting on my bum for long periods of time – and while sitting there exploring the Internet there is nothing nicer than a cup of tea and a sandwich to keep me going. My bum has developed some interesting dimples that I have not seen in a number of years and my tum some fascinating rolls of fat.

Finding the solution to all this is really not difficult, and the same applies to me as to anyone else. Do not blame age and give up: poor lifestyle is the culprit. Change those habits and create new, active, healthy lifestyle patterns, and you will find a huge difference in the way you look and feel no matter what your age.

With the right frame of mind and the perfect combination of a little knowledge the aim of this book is to provide you, realistically, with the tools to help bring about the changes you want, resulting in a shape to your tum and bum that is ageless. It is never too late, and you are never too old, to take control and combat the excesses that take their toll around your middle and your rear. With a little knowledge, practice and effort, you can make a real difference to your tum and bum, in just 10 minutes a day. The effects of physical exercise and increased body awareness mean that you will look better and you will start to become more conscious of feeling better too. This in turn results in raised self-esteem and a renewed motivation to keep going to achieve complete success, not just in body shaping but in other areas of your life.

I hope you will enjoy practising the exercises, which are favourites from my classes. I would also urge you to read all the chapters, especially Chapter 6 on Posture, which is the foundation for everything that follows, and remember to use the visualisation exercise provided in Chapter 5 – It's All in Your MInd. Above all, have fun.

it is never too late and you are never to old to take control and combat the excesses that take their toll around your middle and your rear what is your

body
shape?

body shape

Traditionally, the human body shape has been divided into three clear categories: **endomorph**, round with large proportions; **ectomorph**, lean with more narrow proportions; and **mesomorph**, wide shoulders and powerful hips with muscular proportions. Studies on body types based on hormonal and hereditary factors have added one more body shape to the above: **the classic 'pear' shape**. But essentially, our bodies tend towards being fat, lean or muscled, and it's the inherited combination of these that influences your shape.

You may not be a perfect match to any of these descriptions, simply because we are all unique, all of us different shapes and sizes; you may even be a combination. However, whether you are short, tall or medium height, you are likely to find that your body shape resembles one of the following.

hip and thigh fat

A woman with this shape has narrow shoulders, a small waist and wide hips. She will have a tendency to put on weight around the lower half of her body below the belly button, particularly on her bum and around her hips and thighs. Excess fat in this body shape leads to lower-level obesity – and hip and thigh fat is harder to shift than upper-body fat.

upper body fat

A woman with this body shape has a more athletic build. She has a strong-looking skeleton with firm limbs that appear muscular, wide shoulders and neck, and strong, powerful hips and buttocks. More masculine in shape, a woman of this body type makes an excellent athlete as she will have more muscle mass than fat tissue. However, poor lifestyle habits will lead to excess weight around her middle. Although it is easier to lose than lower-level fat, abdominal fat is associated with high blood pressure and heart disease.

top to toe fat

A woman with this body shape has been chubby since childhood. Her bone structure is average to large with a thickset frame, and her hips and shoulders are wide. She is generally unsporty, and when she puts on weight it is all over her body rather than just in one place – her excesses appear on both lower and upper body. She will have a life-long battle with her weight if she is not careful with her eating habits and exercise.

not a lot of fat

A woman with this body shape is the lucky one in today's world, as she fits the blueprint of what is beautiful. She has a small to average bone structure; her bones are long and slender, with long arms and legs in relation to her trunk. Her musculature is slight. She has a metabolism like a racehorse and carries very little excess body fat.

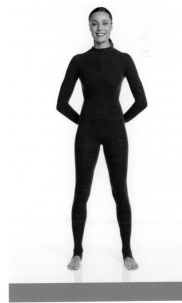

Once you have established your shape, you need to recognise and accept that this is the body that you were born with and there is nothing you can do to change its basic structure. There is, however, an enormous amount you can do to make the best of the shape that you have, and this book will show you how to begin that process by targeting your bum and tum.

13

about your

tum & bum

your tum

Our fascination with our tum and bum is centred on their shape, tone and the amount of fat surrounding them. That fascination is heavily influenced by **society's image of what is attractive** and what is not, and we therefore strive to achieve the perfect image – sometimes unrealistically. While image is important to how we feel about ourselves, it is also important to realise that the areas we have targeted have a function in everyday life. **The first step towards achieving a perfect tum and bum** is to develop an awareness that both areas play an important role in posture and movement.

the spine

The spinal column (or your backbone) is made up of a number of vertebrae that start at the neck and end at the tailbone. These vertebrae are moulded into different groups each with a different function and shape and size. Starting at the neck is the cervical spine, which is designed to be flexible for movement of the head. Less flexible are the thoracic vertebrae, which make up most of the spine and are responsible for twisting rotational movements. Those that make up the lower back are the lumbar vertebrae. These are larger, thicker, wider bones whose job it is to support and balance the upper body. At the bottom of the spine is the sacrum, a wedge-shaped bone that attaches to the pelvic girdle to provide a stable base for the spinal column. Last comes the coccyx, which is your tailbone.

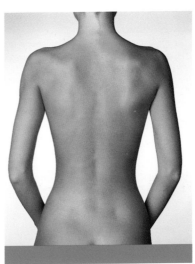

The vertebrae are stacked on top of each other like building blocks, but they are not straight. They make an 'S' shape, curving in at the neck and lower back and slightly out in the middle of the thoracic vertebrae. This is simply because if your spine was straight then during movement – especially running and jumping – shock would be transmitted through the body. That 'S' shape acts as a shock absorber, preventing the spine from being shaken or jarred.

Each vertebra is separated from its neighbour by a spongy disc, which is attached to the vertebrae above and below. Each disc is made up of a hard outer case and a spongy gel on the inside. With age and inactivity the disc gel begins to dry up and the spine becomes less flexible, so it is essential to remain active. Discs can degenerate and are heavily influenced by a number of factors including age, lifestyle, the way you move and your state of mind. Exercise can slow this degenerative process by improving mobility and flexibility in the joints. It can also increase circulation and strengthen the muscles that hold the spine in place. Did you know that you are taller in the morning than in the evening? This is because the discs between the vertebrae are thicker before you wake up, before the effects of gravity and poor lifestyle habits set in. We get shorter as we get older, because the discs between our vertebrae shrink.

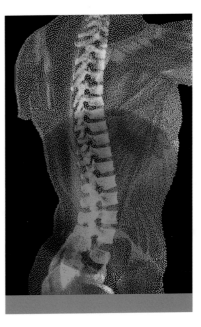

17

Spinal Alignment

Because the spine consists of vertebrae stacked one on top of the other like building blocks, if some of those building blocks are out of alignment the spine will become unstable, placing stress and strain on the joints, ligaments and muscles. One of the aims of the 10-minute tone-up exercise programme in this book is to promote good posture, by training the lumbar spine to be aligned in a 'neutral' position and the muscles and tissues surrounding it to be at their normal length.

the abdominal muscles

The abdominal muscles are like a natural corset for the body. They act to stabilise the spine and support the internal organs; they also allow movement – bending forwards and sideways and twisting and rotating.

the straight abdominal muscle

The abdominals are made up of three layers of muscle which run in different directions. In the outer, or superficial, layer and in the centre of the abdomen is the straight abdominal muscle, the rectus abdominus. It works to bend the spine forwards and sideways, and is also known as the 'six-pack' abdominal muscle, as it has a rippled effect on very lean, toned, well-muscled people.

the muscles of the waist

On each side of the abdomen are two muscles that run diagonally. The outer layer is the external oblique, the second layer the internal oblique. The primary function of these muscle groups is to rotate the spine and allow us to bend over sideways. They also help other abdominal muscle groups.

the deep abdominal muscles

Under the obliques and in the third and deepest layer of the abdominal wall is the transverse abdominal muscle group. It is now recognised that this group is crucial to the stability of the lumbar spine. It is not connected with movement other than to hold the tummy in. The transverse also plays an important role in holding the contents of your tummy in when you cough or sneeze.

In any movement that involves the abdominals, most of the muscles will be used. Curling up with your shoulders off the floor will use the upper part of the straight abdominal muscle. Tilting the pelvis with your legs off the floor will work the lower part. Any twisting movements will involve the obliques, while pulling the abdominals in tight will activate the transverse.

A successful exercise programme works both the superficial and deep abdominal muscles by improving their strength and endurance. Once you start to achieve this, you will find that your tummy muscles will look and feel tighter and flatter and your posture will improve.

your bum

Modern-day living means we are **less active then we should be**. We have jobs where we are seated all day, we drive instead of walking, we sit and watch television or spend hours at a computer. The result is excess weight and slack muscles around our rear end. The buttock muscles are responsible for the shape of your bum; they also have a major influence on your posture and movement. The key to a **more toned, leaner bum** is to recognise the role that these muscles play. You can do this by developing an understanding of the muscles that pass over the hip joint.

the pelvis

The pelvic girdle is formed by the two hip bones and the wedge-shaped bone in the middle called the sacrum. A woman's pelvis is generally wider than a man's because she is built to give birth, so the width of her hips has to allow room for the birth canal. The function of the pelvic girdle is to provide support and protection for the internal organs and to connect the torso and the legs. The hip joint is a ball-and-socket joint, which means that it is flexible and can move in almost every direction.

Take a moment to explore just what your hip joints can do. Gently swing your leg forwards, backwards and sideways, then rotate it inwards and outwards.

the buttock and outer thigh muscles

As we are targeting the bum area, the main muscles we are concerned with are those that surround and cross the hip joint. These are the main buttock muscles, the gluteus maximus and gluteus medius, and the small buttock muscle, the gluteus minimus. All of these are attached to the pelvis and play an important role in dynamic movement and posture.

The gluteus maximus is one of the largest muscles in the body. It is responsible for powerful movements, extending the leg backwards, and it also rotates the thigh outwards. The gluteus maximus forms the shape of your buttocks and you use it when you climb the stairs, stand up from a sitting position or jump up and down.

Underneath the gluteus maximus are the gluteus medius and gluteus minimus. Despite being called the outer thigh or abductor muscles, these muscles are situated high on the hipbone and they work to take your leg out sideways away from the midline of your body. They are activated by walking and running, and play an important role in supporting and stabilising the hip joint during movement, when it bears a lot of force.

the **hip** and **inner thigh** muscles

Although the 10-minute tone-ups in this book focus primarily on the muscles of your bum, you need to ensure you have an exercise programme that will balance all your muscle groups. The function of the muscles is to provide support and stability to the skeleton, and unbalanced muscles not only affect your shape but can create postural problems. For a well-rounded exercise programme, you need to work opposing muscle groups; for example, if you work your outer thigh you also need to work your inner thigh. When you work your buttock muscles, you also need to pay attention to their opposite muscle group, the hip flexors.

You can feel your hip flexors in the crease at the top of your leg, or when you bring your knees towards your chest. These muscles work when you bend at the hip, for example when climbing the stairs. Often they become short and tight and this may affect your posture. Stretching your hip flexors is an important part of your exercise programme.

The inner thigh muscles have the opposite effect to the abductors, working to bring your legs into and past the midline of your body. Generally stronger than the outer thighs, this muscle group tends to become flabby with lack of use and is often targeted for toning. This is also the muscle group responsible for groin strain in sports such as horse riding and ice skating. Regular stretching and strength work can help you avoid these injuries.

The hip rotators are a small group of muscles that wrap around the hip joint. Along with the buttock muscles, the hip rotators control the rotational movement when you walk. You are constantly using this group of muscles: every time you turn a corner or change direction you use them. If your hip rotators become over-tight they will inhibit all your turning movements. These muscles are generally used when you work other muscle groups.

for a well-rounded exercise programme, you need to work with opposing muscle groups

21

3

how fit are

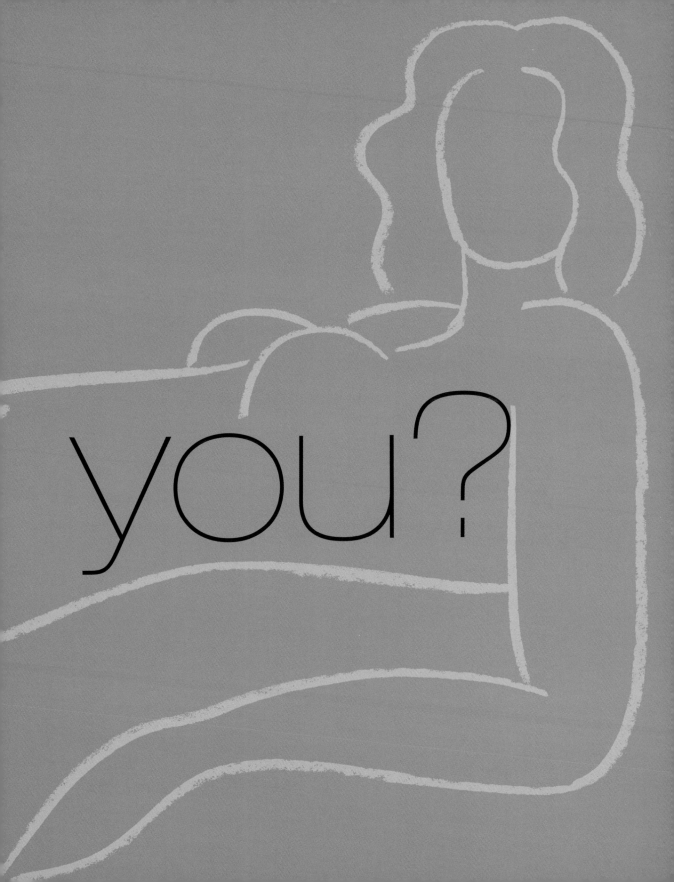

you?

how fit are you?

The type of exercise you need to focus on for your tum and bum is **strength and endurance work**. The aim is to improve both of these in your abdominal and buttock muscles, for a **toned look and better posture** and body alignment, and of course to develop greater endurance for everyday living. You can do this by being very clear about how to work your muscles in both ways.

strength and endurance

Strength is often defined as the maximum amount of force a muscle can produce to overcome a resistance: the image that comes to mind is the 'strongest man in the world' pulling along a bus or lifting an exceptionally heavy weight. Strength training means applying progressive force to stimulate your muscles into becoming stronger and more sculpted-looking.

Endurance is the muscles' ability to produce force over and over again: think of a marathon runner. You develop endurance by supplying blood to the muscles through repetitive movements, which results in burned calories and a more toned look.

For your 10-minute tone-ups you need to use a combination of the two types of exercise, because gains in strength help to enhance endurance. With a good combination of strength and endurance you can really make the most of your tum and bum.

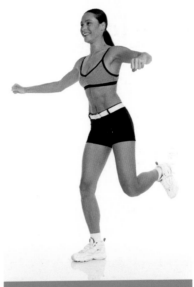

Working Your Muscles

The muscles surrounding your skeleton are the body's support system – without them you would collapse in a heap. Your muscles are made up of muscle fibres that are attached to your bones, which act as levers around the joint. Movement is brought about through the motor nerves that are attached to these muscle fibres. When your brain sends a message down the nerve, the muscle fibres attached to that particular nerve will contract; when your muscles contract, they pull on the bone and you move.

The amount of force you want to use in your muscles will determine how many muscle fibres you use. So, if you make only a half-hearted effort when exercising your tum and bum you won't use as many muscle fibres as you would if you put in more effort, and the result will be less muscle tone. You need to work as many muscle fibres as possible to stimulate the muscles to become stronger and more toned, and this is achieved through progression and variety in your exercise routine.

25

the right way

To achieve a strong, toned bum and tum you need to train them regularly. As your exercise programme is limited to 10 minutes a day, you must make sure that every time you work your muscles your training session is effective.

muscles and metabolism

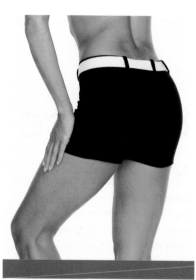

The rate at which you burn calories is called your metabolism. Your metabolic rate changes over the course of your lifetime and is influenced by many different factors.

Your body type plays an important role in your rate of calorie burning. A more muscular person is likely to burn more calories than a fat person, as muscle is more metabolically active than fat, so people with more muscle mass than fat mass will burn more calories. Men come into this category because they generally have more muscle mass than women do, but women who have a muscular body type are more likely to have a higher metabolic rate than those with round or pear-shaped bodies that are prone to putting on weight quickly. Your height and weight will affect the rate at which you burn energy: a taller, heavier person will burn more calories than a shorter, lighter person.

Lastly, age affects metabolism. The metabolic rate of the body peaks at around the age of 20 and begins to decline thereafter. At around 30 muscle mass starts to decline, and as this happens body fat starts to increase so that you put on weight, particularly around your tum and bum. You can, however, combat this ageing process, as it is actually not so much age but poor lifestyle habits and lack of exercise that take their toll on your metabolism.

If you become inactive and don't use your muscles, you will find that they decrease in size and lose shape, and your metabolism will start to slow down. Remember, the more muscle you have the more calories you will burn, so the way to increase your metabolic rate is to increase your muscle mass through regular exercise.

age affects metabolism. The metabolic rate of the body peaks at around the age of 20 and begins to decline thereafter

The combination of aerobic work and strength training will enable you to increase your metabolic rate, keeping your body fat low and stimulating your muscles into growing bigger and stronger, thereby giving them a more toned, sculpted shape.

balance in exercise

Your muscles pull – they do not push. Just imagine curling your wrist up to your shoulder: the bicep is pulling the forearm to the shoulder. If you want to straighten your arm again, your brain gives the opposite group, the triceps, the signal to pull on the bone and extend the arm. Your muscles work together in pairs: when one muscle contracts, its opposite relaxes, just as in the biceps curl.

The same goes for the muscles that you will be focusing on in your 10-minute tone-ups, the abdominal and buttock muscles. As you curl forwards, the abdominal muscles contract and shorten while the muscles in your back lengthen to allow the movement. With your buttock muscles, as you extend your leg behind you the muscles of your bottom contract while their opposite, the hip flexors, lengthen.

How you train your muscles will be reflected in how they develop, so it is very important to be aware of the potential hazards involved in training individual muscle groups. The problem with targeting specific muscles is that you tend to forget their opposites. Doing too much of one exercise can create imbalance elsewhere; for example, over a period of time working only the abdominals and not including the back muscles will result in the abdominals becoming shorter and tighter while leaving the back muscles long and weak. This can alter the alignment of the body, creating an out-of-proportion look and potential postural problems that may end up as injury at a later stage. We will be looking at opposite muscles in greater detail in Chapter 6 on Posture.

No Bulky Muscles

Very often women misunderstand strength work, thinking that if they apply resistance to their muscles they will bulk up like a man. As a result, time is often wasted doing endless repetitions of an exercise with little or no resistance, which causes frustration because the outcome is little gain in muscle tone and not a lot of change in body shape. Such exercise will burn few calories and eventually cause wear and tear to your joints.

In fact, it is highly unlikely that a woman will bulk up like a man. Women have less muscle mass than men and 10 times less testosterone, so unless you are in training for body-building or taking stimulants it will be difficult for

27

you to bulk up in this way. However, while you may not grow bulky-looking muscles, strength training does increase tone, to give a more sculpted look by making your muscles appear denser. Unlike men, women can double their strength without gaining in muscle size. On the other hand, if you tone up but are covered in layers of excess body fat, then there is a possibility that you will look bulky. You need to lose the body fat so that your muscles will appear lean and toned underneath.

To make the most of your 10 minutes of toning, you need a strength programme that places progressive resistance on your muscles so that they will become toned and strong and remain this way throughout your life, keeping you looking good and feeling fit for longer.

Overload: Stronger for Longer

When you 'overload' your muscles, you challenge them by working them harder than you ordinarily would do on a day-to-day basis. You do this by applying progressive force to stimulate your muscles into becoming stronger and more toned. As this happens, they will take longer to tire and you will be able to recover more quickly from one exercise to another. You will also find that your movements will become smoother and more co-ordinated.

To achieve this progression safely and effectively, it is essential that you work at the correct level. If you do too little exercise, you will achieve minimal results; if you work too hard or too quickly, you could end up injured. Endless repetitions of an exercise may not give you the firmer shape you desire and can also take their toll on your body.

Challenge Your Muscles

To become firmer you need to challenge your muscles to work longer and harder. Increasing the intensity of your workout, or lengthening the time, or increasing the number of exercise days per week are the ways to achieve this successfully.

For example, you may start by doing five repetitions of an exercise, and then when this becomes easy you could increase that to seven. When that becomes easy go to 10. Once you have built up to, say, 20, you then need to ask yourself how you can overload your muscles some more without doing endless repetitions. If you were to continue to 30, 40 or even 50 repetitions you would be exerting the same amount of force for a longer period, thereby increasing your endurance.

For a firmer-looking tum and bum, you would need to stop at 20 repetitions and then challenge the muscles some more by increasing the intensity or changing the type of exercise that you do. For the 10-minute tone-ups in this book, we have increased the intensity and varied the exercises.

Muscle Fatigue

When your muscles are becoming overloaded during the last repetitions of an exercise, they start to become fatigued. It may feel very difficult to perform another repetition, or your muscles may feel tired and weak or depleted of energy. You may get a burning sensation in the area that you are working, which is caused by the build-up of a waste product called lactic acid. This is absolutely normal and as soon as you stop exercising you will find that it goes away, metabolised and recycled by the body.

Some muscles become fatigued more quickly than others, especially if you are not used to working them. You may find this with your abdominal and buttock muscles. Muscle soreness for a few days following exercise is also fairly common. It is caused by tiny tears in the connective tissues that hold the muscles together and some tearing of the membrane of the muscle cells. If you are so sore and stiff that you can hardly move, then you have done too much too soon. You need to slow down and work at a level that is comfortable but still challenging.

exercise technique

When you start to exercise, pay particular attention to the concentration and visualisation techniques on pages 58–59. The quality of your exercise routine is far more important than the quantity of exercises that you perform. Time restrictions in our lives often cause us to rush, trying to get as many things as we can done in as little time as possible, and this is often the way with exercise too.

Speed

For effective work on your abdominal and buttock muscles, performing each exercise at the correct speed is very important. Fast, jerky actions can restrict your range of movement and place strain on the joints as well as reduce their flexibility. To be safe but effective in your exercise routine you need to work slowly and smoothly through the full range of motion.

To achieve quality movements in your tum and bum exercises, the actions need to be performed slowly and in a controlled manner in both directions. For example, when you do a curl-up (see page 85) you lift your shoulders for 2 counts and lower back down for 2 to 4 counts.

Practice

For the complete beginner it is best to start with minimum resistance but lots of practice, performing each exercise slowly both ways. At the beginning, developing awareness of how an exercise should feel is essential, because it is when you are learning that you fix the habits that you then carry through into every exercise session you do.

It is also helpful to know which way your muscles move, so that you can work on fine-tuning your quality of movement. For example, you know that your obliques run diagonally on either side of the straight abdominal wall, so the movement to practise for this muscle group is diagonally from one shoulder towards the opposite hip bone.

Correct Positioning

Putting your body in the correct position is also essential when working your abdominal and buttock muscles, as starting off with poor exercise posture or having your pelvis tilted the wrong way will place undue strain on your joints and affect your musculature. Standing with straight legs and knees locked, for example, can result in the pelvis tilting forwards, which forces the back to curve past its natural line. Starting with a neutral spine is very important. Remember: the way you train your muscles will determine the way in which they develop.

Breathing

The breath plays an important role in exercise. Slow, controlled breathing keeps you relaxed and eases tension in both mind and body so that they work as one. As you do your tum and bum exercises, aim to exhale when you do the movement that requires the effort and inhale on the return movement.

Sets and Reps

Exercises to condition specific muscle groups are usually performed in sets and reps (repetitions) to achieve best results in a muscle. The number of repetitions in an exercise is the number of times you repeat a movement, and this is continued until your muscles are overloaded. Sets of an exercise are a group of repetitions. The aim for the 10-minute tone-ups is not to perform a specific number of repetitions, but to work within guidelines until your muscles feel tired. At the end of each set of repetitions your muscles should feel fatigued – this shows that they have been successfully over-loaded. If you feel nothing at the end of a set of tum or bum exercises, then you have not worked hard enough and will need to look at different ways to overload your muscles.

Research suggests that you get the same increases in strength and muscle tone by doing one set of an exercise as you do by doing two or three sets, as long as the set you do is of maximum quality. This method is effective, and great if you have limited time available. My personal experience is that doing two sets of an exercise is more beneficial than doing one, the advantages being that you achieve better muscle strength and tone and burn more calories. So, when you have reached a level within the 10-minute tone-up programme where you can do all the exercises with ease in one set, you need to progress to two sets and start splitting your routine.

Take a Break

One of the great things about 10-minute tone-ups is that you can focus on working just one muscle group each day. This is a most beneficial way to exercise, because it is actually very important not to work the same muscle group hard for two days running. While it is fine to do different aerobic activities every day, it is not advisable to perform resistance exercises on the same muscle group day after day. This is because resistance training exhausts your muscles and they need time to recover, and this takes place the following day, when the muscles are rebuilding and strengthening. A really good way of working out is to focus on your tum one day and your bum the next, so that each

working just one muscle group a day is a beneficial way to exercise

muscle group has a day off in between. To achieve the best results from toning your bum and tum, you need to make sure you exercise each muscle group two to three times a week.

It also helps to take a small rest in between sets of an exercise if your muscles are feeling particularly tired. Stretching the muscle group you have just worked is relaxing, takes tightness out of a muscle and returns it to its original length.

The following exercise is one you can do if you want a short rest during or following an abdominal exercise.

Lie on your back with your feet on the floor and your knees bent. Raise your buttocks off the floor and hold for 4 counts, then lower for 4 counts. This relaxes your abdominals, allowing blood to flow back to the area. It also works your bum.

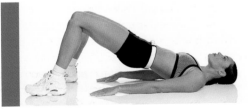

31

flexibility

While the focus for our 10-minute tone-ups is strength and endurance work, it is important to consider the other principles of fitness so that your body is well balanced. Doing too much of one type of exercise can pull your body out of alignment and result in injury. For example, your muscles may become stronger and more toned, but if they are not supple they are likely to pull or strain more easily. The muscles you are focusing on are the abdominal and buttock muscles, both of which play an important role in posture. If these muscles become too tight through toning they will be out of balance with the rest of your body, and this could have a major effect on your posture.

For the 10-minute tone-up programme, strength work and flexibility exercises make a perfect combination for the tum and bum. As well as tightening these areas through strength and endurance work, you also need to relax your muscles by stretching them.

You are supple when your joints are able to move freely through their full range of motion. Suppleness is individual and is influenced by a number of factors. Genetics plays an important role in determining your flexibility – some people are naturally more supple than others. Gender also has an effect on suppleness: on the whole, men are less flexible than women. This is because women are designed for a greater range of flexibility in the pelvic region to facilitate childbirth.

Age also influences how supple you are, for we tend to lose flexibility as we grow older. But the factor that has the most marked effect on how flexible you are is your lifestyle. The stresses and tensions of everyday life inevitably take their toll on the body, creating tightness and stiffness in the limbs and joints.

Flexibility and Exercise

The exercises you do will have an effect on your suppleness. If you tone your muscles but don't stretch them, you will decrease the range of movement at a joint. Your muscles may also start to look short and tight.

Flexibility is an important part of an exercise regime. You stretch to warm up and prepare your muscles and joints for the exercise ahead, and you do this by lengthening the muscles to increase their range of movement and improve circulation around the joints. You stretch at the end of an exercise session to lengthen out the tightened muscles you have just worked, to maintain and develop your flexibility so that your body can become looser and so that you can work more efficiently through an increased range of movement. It has also been suggested that stretching after exercise minimises muscle soreness.

Lastly, stretching is highly beneficial because it relaxes your muscles and reduces tension in both body and mind.

The Stretch Reflex

You become more flexible by lengthening your muscles so that movement is increased around a joint. To prevent your muscles from over-stretching, the stretch reflex comes into play. This mechanism works by sending a signal to the spinal cord, which returns with an order to the muscle to contract to protect it from injury. If you stretch too quickly or with jerky, bouncing movements, the contraction can be more forceful and injury can occur.

As you stretch, tension develops in your muscles. If you hold a stretch for long enough (around 20 seconds), a point is reached where the tension disappears and your muscles can be stretched even further.

if you hold a stretch for long enough, tension disappears and you can stretch further

You can stretch any time, any place, as long as the environment is warm: stretching cold, tight muscles is more likely to end in injury. Stretching in the bath or shower is relaxing, as your muscles will be warm and pliable. When you go into each stretch, you need to do so carefully and slowly. In exercise, it is advisable to raise your body temperature to ensure that your muscles are pliable before placing any tension on them; you can do this by moving on the spot until you feel warm.

Ballistic Stretching

Ballistic stretching involves fast, jerking, bouncing movements, which encourage the stretch reflex to be more forceful. It has been suggested that this type of stretching is beneficial for specific sports where dynamic flexibility is needed to copy particular actions in the sport. However, most experts agree that stretching with repeated jerky, bouncing movements is the least beneficial technique for the general population and can increase the risk of injury.

Static Stretching

The preferred method of stretching is called static stretching, which is a gentle, gradual stretch in a held position for a period of time. With this type of stretching, the stretch reflex is slow and mild and the muscle is given time to relax and lengthen further.

For the 10-minute tone-ups you need to focus on stretching the particular muscle groups that you are toning. For the warm-up (see Chapter 7) you might want to incorporate stretching to make your muscles more pliable. When you are performing warm-up or maintenance stretches, hold each one for at least 8 to 10 seconds. At the end of your workout you may need to work on increasing your flexibility, which you can do through developmental stretching. You can hold these stretches for longer, say 15 to 30 seconds or even longer. As you feel the tension easing in the muscle, you gently increase the stretch. Remember not to jerk or bounce and to hold the stretch still. You should not feel any pain, just tension in the muscle.

33

aerobic exercise for a perfect tum and bum

Toning and stretching alone will not get you a perfect-looking rear or a flatter tummy. If both areas are covered in fat then you may tighten up and become stronger, but your shape will not be that different. For a better shape you need to burn calories to lose the excess fat around those areas. And what is the best way to burn calories? Answer: aerobic exercise.

The last component of fitness that plays an important role in tum and bum shaping is aerobic exercise. Aerobic means requiring oxygen and your aerobic fitness is defined by the ability of your cardiovascular system to deliver oxygen to your working muscles. This type of exercise involves using the major muscles of the body, including those of the buttocks, in large, rhythmic movements to make the body demand a greater volume of oxygen. The heart and lungs have to work to supply that oxygen, and the more you move your muscles the harder the heart has to work in order to meet the demand.

As you progress in exercise, your muscles adapt to the workloads that have been placed upon them by becoming more efficient in extracting oxygen. They become more toned and you burn fat more efficiently, your heartbeat becomes slower and stronger, and you become fitter. These are not the only benefits: aerobic exercise plays an important role in reducing the risk of heart disease and is instrumental in rehabilitating people with heart problems. It has also become part of treatment programmes for conditions like diabetes, high blood pressure and, of course, weight problems.

Controlling Your Body Weight

Your body weight is made up of bones, muscles, organs, fluids and fat. A number of factors affect your weight, including your height and build. A short, stocky woman at her ideal body weight is likely to weigh more than a short woman with a very lean, skinny build.

You could also have two women of the same height and same build, yet one may weigh more. It could be that she has excess body fat, but it is also possible that her muscles are strong and toned because she has done strength work in the gym. As muscle weighs more than fat, she will be heavier, even though she may look better than the woman who weighs less. Often women feel they don't need to exercise because they are the same weight as when they were at school. However, this may be because there is a reduction in total body weight as muscles decrease with age and body fat increases!

When we hop on the bathroom scales in the morning we often assume that the weight we are reading is fat. In fact, the scales cannot tell the difference between fat mass and the rest of our body make-up. What we are really concerned about when we discuss our weight is the amount of fat we have on our bodies. This is far more important than how much we weigh on our bathroom scales, and I would strongly suggest that you throw the latter in the dustbin.

In the past, body weight was often assessed by height-to-weight charts, but these have now proven to be unreliable as they do not take body composition into consideration. A better method of working out your ideal body weight is to find your body mass index (BMI).

Work in metric. Divide your weight in kilograms by the square of your height in metres. So, if your weight is 60kg and your height is 1.65m, you would work to the following equation.

1.65 x 1.65 = 2.7225
60kg divided by 2.7225 = BMI 22

You should aim to keep your body mass index between 19 and 25. Anything less then 19 is underweight, 19 to 25 is normal, between 25 and 29 is overweight. Anything over this is obese.

My own opinion is that your ideal body weight is the weight at which you look and feel your best. You can monitor your body fat levels by seeing how your clothes fit. If they are becoming looser then you are clearly reducing your size. I think the most effective way of checking your progress is to use good old-fashioned girth measurements. You will soon know if you are reducing inches from your bum and tum because the measurements will change.

Ask a friend to measure you and try to get the same person to do it every time. Keep a note of your measurements in a diary and take them again every six to eight weeks. Take two measurements:
1 Tummy: across the level of your belly button;
2 Hips: at the maximum protrusion of your bum.

Fat

Fat makes up a percentage of your body weight and is stored all over the body in fat cells under the skin, in the skeletal muscles and around the internal organs. You need a certain amount of fat to protect your internal organs, to insulate you and as a reserve fuel supply. In the old days, in times of famine a woman would call on her fat reserves to feed her young. Fat is needed for survival. However, the body can accumulate endless amounts of it and it is stored in fat cells when not being used. When a person gains weight, fat cells fill up and increase in size and when weight is lost fat cells release fat and reduce in size.

We have already seen that different body types distribute fat in different places (see page 13). Some people carry their excesses around their middle, others around their hips and bum, still others have a more even distribution of body fat on both tum and bum, while some carry very little body fat at all. The hormonal influence on a woman's body means that on the whole she has more fat than a man does. It also means that fat is distributed in different parts of the body at different times in her life. For example, a woman who has stored fat around her hips, thighs and bottom may find that later on in life she puts on weight around her middle. This is because after menopause levels of the hormone oestrogen start to fall, which results in a change of fat distribution from the hips and thighs to the tummy. But whatever stage of life you are at and whatever body type you are, the bottom line is that fat is fat and the only way to get rid of it is through burning calories and a sensible eating plan.

different types of body distribute fat in different places at different times of life

Cellulite

Many women suffer from a 'cottage cheese' effect in certain areas of the body, particularly the rear end – this is called cellulite. It is often suggested that this is a different type of fat, the result of a hormonal imbalance within the fat cells that causes this effect on the hips, thighs and other areas of the body. Another theory is that fat is fat and cellulite arises from the difference between the structure of men's and women's skin and the connective tissue that builds chambers where layers of fat are stored. Whatever the truth of the matter, you can improve the appearance of these problem areas by diet and, of course, exercise.

Spot Reduction

A popular myth is that you can lose fat selectively from one area of your body. The fact is that everyone is different: some people will lose fat from their middle before anywhere else, others lose it from their upper body. It is a well-known fact now that fat around your tummy is easier to lose than fat on your bum. Hip and thigh fat is harder to shift because it is put there for storage. The one way to shift this fat quickly is to breastfeed, and women who choose not to do so are holding back the mechanism that will start to release fat from these areas.

Fat is stored all over the body and when you diet and exercise it is taken from all your fat cells, not just one area. However, you can tone up muscles in one particular area to give you a much firmer shape, and this is exactly what you will be doing in your 10-minute tone-ups.

Burning Calories

To start losing excess body fat around your rear and your middle, you need to boost your metabolism and become more active. Large, rhythmic movements using the large muscles of the body, including the buttock muscles, are needed to make the heart and lungs work harder to generate more oxygen for use in fat metabolism.

The harder or longer you work, the more fat you are burning. As you progress, your fitness levels increase and your body becomes more efficient at burning calories and processing oxygen.

For long-term fat loss, it is consistency in exercise that will make the difference. Although it may often seem that only a small number of calories are burnt in each session, it is the regularity of exercise that will help you make progress. Say you burn 200 calories in a 30-minute aerobic session: if you do the same three times a week, that is 600 calories; over a month it adds up to 2,400 calories, and over a year 28,800. If we work on the basis that 3,500 calories represents about 0.45 kg (1 lb) of fat, then in one year you will have lost 3.7 kg (8 lbs) – and that's without even looking at your diet yet!

Ideally, you need to do aerobic sessions at least three times a week, for at least 20 to 30 minutes each time. However, if you simply don't have the time you can still benefit from doing 10 minutes a day. While the calories burnt may be minimal – say, 50 to 70 – you will still have given your metabolism a boost, have better circulation and tone in your muscles, and, most importantly, feel good, with a degree of improved cardiovascular fitness.

You can also help to boost your metabolism by putting more effort into the things you do on a daily basis. For example, take the stairs instead of the lift, walk wherever you can and do the housework with full gusto – I certainly feel warm and that I have worked my muscles every time I use a vacuum cleaner.

37

for long-term fat loss, consistency in exercise will make the difference

Metabolism Boosters

The following exercises are 10-minute metabolism boosters for the abdominal and buttock muscles.

1 Step up and down on the stairs or an exercise step.

2 For the outer thigh, as you step up take the other leg out to the side and squeeze your buttocks. Make sure you are not just kicking out to the side but are working from the hip. Check that your toes, knees and hips are facing forwards.

3 For the buttock muscles, as you step up take the other leg out behind you and squeeze your buttocks. Make sure that your stepping is slightly soft, with your foot facing forwards. Hold your abdominals in tight and do not arch your back as you take your leg out behind.

For all three exercises, make sure the movement remains smooth, controlled and rhythmic as you change from one leg to the other.

Space hoppers are not only great for children's fitness, you can have a lot of fun on one too. Jumping up and down on a space hopper will give your buttock muscles a great workout and get you out of breath: take my word for it!

Overload

As well as consistency, it is pushing yourself harder than you do ordinarily that will make all the difference to your shape. The same overload principle applies to aerobic work as to working your muscles: to become fitter and start to gain more tone, you need to feel safely challenged. As you become fitter, you need to be challenged some more. This can be done by increasing the intensity of your workout, lengthening the time that you spend on it or increasing the number of times you exercise.

There are several different ways of monitoring the intensity of your workout. Heart-rate monitoring watches are very useful, though expensive; taking your pulse can also help. But I believe the most effective heart-rate monitor is you! Quite simply, monitoring how you honestly feel is just as good as any scientific method of measuring your heart rate. For example, if you find at the end of 10 minutes that you are not out of breath at all and can very easily hold a conversation, then you have clearly not worked hard enough. On the other hand, if you are so out of breath that you cannot speak at all, then you have worked too hard. But if you are comfortably out of breath then you will know that you have worked well.

Do remember that even if you are working out for only 10 minutes a day, technique is important. Ten minutes of exercising wrongly or too hard can still end up in injury.

remember that even if you are working out for only 10 minutes a day, technique is important

muscles and
pregnancy

Pregnancy can make big demands on your waistline – it can increase from, say, 65 cm (25 in) to 115 cm (45 in). As pregnancy progresses, the developing baby throws your body weight forward, and you make up for this by leaning back. This results in a change in posture by exaggerating the spinal curves, which can place a lot of strain on your lower back. In addition, in order to adapt to the growing baby your abdominals must stretch. These muscles stretch lengthways. Meanwhile, sideways stretching is caused by the splitting of the fibrous tissue that joins the two parts of the straight abdominal muscle together. This split is called a 'diastasis'.

Abdominal exercise is most important during pregnancy in order to strengthen the weakened abdominal wall, reduce any strain on the lower back and correct any postural faults that may occur. However, it is also essential that no undue strain be placed on these areas, as too much strong abdominal work can cause doming of the abdominal wall. A tum that sticks out like this is not only unsightly but also denotes weakness in the abdominal muscles, which can have an effect on posture and the lower back.

Another consideration is how you do your abdominal exercise. Sometimes in the later stages of pregnancy lying on your back is not advised (check with your doctor). This is because the weight of the baby can press on the main blood vessels, which may compress them and reduce the blood supply to the heart and other organs.

▶ tummy tightener

Sit tall on the edge of a solid chair with your feet comfortably apart. Place one hand on your tum and the other on your lower back. Practise pulling your tummy in to tighten the abdominal muscles. Hold for 2 counts and gently release. You can actually do this exercise while standing, sitting or lying, at any time and in any place.

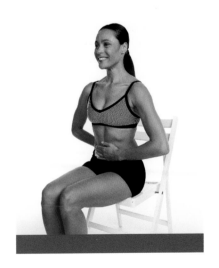

make sure you breathe naturally and normally and check that you are not slouching

39

▶ pelvic tilt

Kneel on all fours with your back straight. Make sure your hands are directly under your shoulders and your knees under your hips, with your feet on the floor. Now tilt your pelvis back towards your heels. Tighten the lower part of your abdominals upwards and in, to draw the baby in towards your spine. Hold for 2 counts and gently release. Avoid arching your back when you release. Feel your spine lengthening.

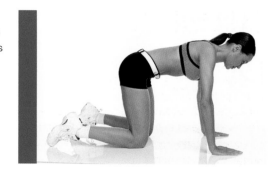

make sure you are breathing naturally and normally; do not hold your breath; ensure your head is comfortably in line with the rest of your body

▶ waist tightener

Kneel on all fours with your back straight. Make sure your hands are directly under your shoulders and your knees under your hips, with your feet on the floor. Now pull the baby in towards your spine and gently tilt your pelvis to the right. At the same time look over your right shoulder. Feel your ribs and the top of your pelvis moving towards each other. Gently come back to the centre. Do the same on the left side. Make sure that your movements are smooth and controlled.

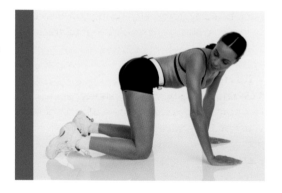

check that the only parts of your body that are moving are your head, ribs and pelvis; breathe naturally and normally

after the birth

In most women, the abdominal muscles gradually begin to join together a few days after the birth. But if the mother has not trained her abdominals after a previous pregnancy, has had a large baby or has carried out strong abdominal exercise, then there is a possibility that her abdominals will not join at the centre and she will develop a 'pendulous abdomen' or big tummy.

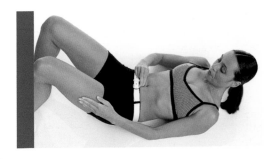

You can check if your tummy muscles have come together by doing the two-finger test. Lie on your back with your knees bent and feet flat on the floor. Raise your head off the ground as if to do a curl-up. Take two fingers and place them just below your tummy button. If there is a hole wider than two fingers then your abdominals have not come together yet. In this case, you need to train them to join back together again and should avoid strong abdominal exercise until this occurs.

The aim for post-natal mums is to condition the abdominals back to pre-pregnancy condition, and to ensure the stability of the spine and encourage good posture. Continue to do the above antenatal exercises plus those below, before embarking on more strenuous abdominal exercise.

▶ head raise

1 Lie on your back with your knees bent and feet comfortably apart. Place a pillow under your head. Pull your tummy in and tuck in your chin. Place your hands on the tops of your thighs.

2 Now raise your head off the pillow to look at your knees. Hold for 1 count and gently lower your head back on to the pillow. Gradually hold the raised position for longer as your abdominals start to become stronger.

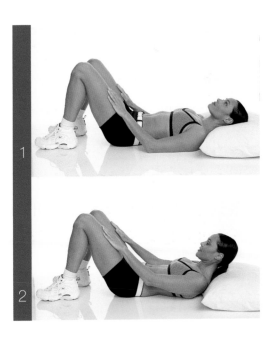

make sure your abdominals remain flat and in control

41

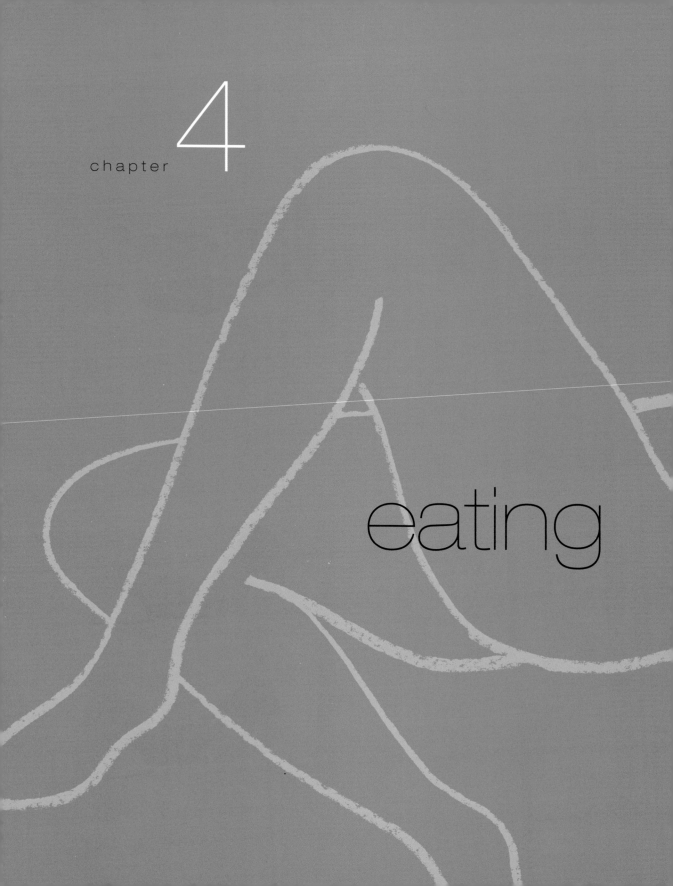

chapter 4

eating

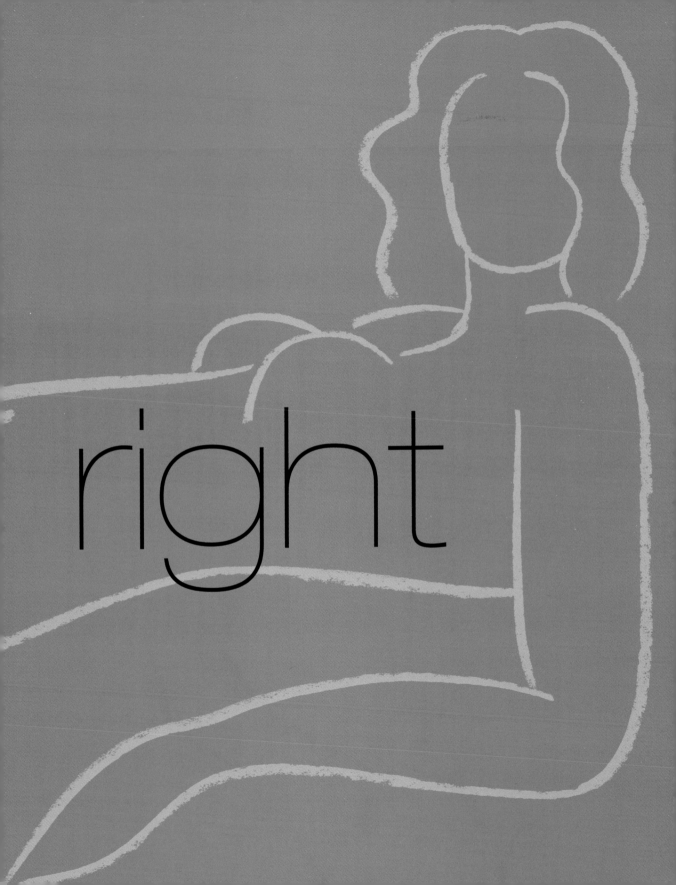

right

eating right

The food you eat has a role to play in the excess fat you carry on your tum and bum. Just as you now have a balanced exercise regime for both areas, you also need to **consider whether your eating habits are balanced.** Abdominal fat can be dangerous to your health, as it is released into the bloodstream more easily than fat from the cells in other parts of your body. This can result in problems for the heart and circulatory system. Together, **exercise and healthy eating** will keep the fat around your tum and bum to a healthy minimum. I would strongly recommend that, in addition to reading this chapter, you consult a book that gives you more detail about your dietary needs.

We all process food differently. Some people need more of a certain type of food than others. Some people can eat as much as they want without putting on weight; others put weight on easily. While keeping this individuality in mind, **the following guidelines for healthy eating** apply to everyone. Your body needs different types of foods to supply the tissues with the nutrients they need. These foods are divided into three categories: carbohydrates, proteins and fats.

food types

Carbohydrates

Carbohydrates supply the body with its primary source of energy and are subdivided into two types: simple sugars and complex carbohydrates.

• **simple sugars** These come in the form of syrup, honey, cane sugar, glucose, treacle, maltose, fructose, malt and molasses. Some of these are found naturally in foods – for example, fruits contain fructose – but most simple sugars are used to improve both the texture and taste of food and to preserve it. Simple sugars are often called 'empty calories' because they provide energy but no other nutrients. When the energy consumed is not used by the body, it is stored as fat. Foods high in simple sugars include cakes and biscuits, sweets, sweetened drinks, sugar-coated cereals and chocolate.

• **refined complex carbohydrates** These types of carbohydrate have been stripped of their nutrients, so that they are reduced to empty calories. These foods include white bread, polished rice and pasta made with refined white flour.

• **complex carbohydrates** In most third-world countries obesity does not exist, because the diet is often very high in complex carbohydrates – the preferred fuel for the body. This type of carbohydrate comes in the form of whole-grain pasta, bread, rice and cereals, vegetables and some fruits. These foods also contain fibre, vitamins and minerals, so are particularly nutritious. Experts suggest that 60 to 65 per cent of the diet should consist of complex carbohydrates.

Fibre

An important part of the diet, fibre is found in plant foods and comes from the plant cell walls. It is not a food group as such: its job is to push food through the digestive system. There are two types of fibre – soluble and insoluble. We need both. Soluble fibre dissolves easily in water and is partly broken down during digestion; all types of fruits and vegetables, pulses, and oats, barley and rye contain soluble fibre. Insoluble fibre is found in bread and pasta, cereals and some vegetables.

Fibre in the diet plays an important role in maintaining good health, by reducing digestive disorders and lowering the incidence of bowel cancer, high blood pressure and constipation. For weight control, fibre – especially the soluble type – helps by filling you up quickly.

Proteins

Protein plays a major role in our bodies. Present in every cell, especially in muscles, it forms the basic building blocks of the body and is responsible for the growth and repair of the body's tissues. Protein is less important when it comes to the provision of energy, for which carbohydrates are the best source.

Proteins are made up from chemicals called amino acids that are found in both animals and plants. There are 20 amino acids in the human body, 12 of which can be manufactured by the body itself. The other eight that cannot are called essential amino acids and must come from the diet. Protein foods include poultry, meat, fish, eggs and cheese, soya, peanuts and pulses.

Experts suggest that 12 per cent of our calories should come from proteins. Most people eat too much, with the excess being stored as fat, resulting in weight gain. Excess protein can also affect your liver and kidneys and cause dehydration.

Fats

Fats are the most concentrated source of energy that we consume and perform a number of roles, including supplying insulation to our bodies and protection for our internal organs. Fat in the diet provides the vitamins A, D, E and K – these can only be obtained by eating foods containing some fat. Fats are also needed to form hormones, which are essential for a vast range of bodily functions, including sexual activity. Finally, fat is a necessary source of energy that can be stored in copious amounts throughout the body.

About 30 per cent of the calories we take in should come from fats, but more often than not we consume more without even realising it. Excess fat in the diet can cause all kinds of health problems including diabetes and obesity, and recently it has been discovered that excess abdominal fat is linked to heart disease – even more reason to strive for a lean tum!

Fats are divided into two groups: saturated fats and unsaturated fats.

● **saturated fats** These are solid at room temperature and animal in origin: the butter on your bread and the fat on your Sunday roast are saturated fats. A little saturated fat in your diet does you no harm, but if taken in excess it can end up increasing blood cholesterol levels and is linked to the potential health problems mentioned above.

● **unsaturated fats** These are divided into two groups: polyunsaturated and monounsaturated. These are the better source of fat to consume in your diet, especially if they are unrefined. These fats are softer at room temperature and can be found in vegetable and fish oils.

For a leaner tum and bum you need to combine exercise with a low-fat diet. The following guidelines will help you to begin reducing fats in your diet.

cut down on
- fried foods
- full-fat cream
- butter and lard
- milk and mayonnaise
- processed meats

(use skimmed milk and light mayonnaise)

47

- oily dressings
- cakes and biscuits
- full-fat cheese (use low-fat)
- fatty meat (trim off fat before cooking)

Look at the labels on the food you buy and always check the fat and sugar content, especially in sauces.

eat more complex carbohydrates and fibre

- pasta, rice, potatoes and bread (unrefined)
- whole grains such as oats, rye, wheat, barley, millet and buckwheat
- vegetables
- fresh fruit
- pulses including lentils, soya beans, kidney beans, black-eyed peas, chick peas, etc

eat moderate amounts of protein

- cut down on red meat
- eat more poultry and fish
- eat low-fat cheese
- eat eggs in moderation
- eat more pulses (as above)

Alcohol

You can also take in empty calories by consuming too much alcohol. Often overlooked in a weight-loss programme, alcohol is very high in calories and too much of it over a period of time can affect your weight, liver and brain, depleting your body of vital vitamins and minerals, and raising your cholesterol levels. Like most things in life, alcohol is something to consume in moderation. Here are a few tips to help you control and reduce your alcohol intake.

- Have a bottle of water on the table at all times
- Choose beer that is low in alcohol
- Drink slowly
- Keep a check on others topping up your glass

Water

Water is fundamental to our existence. Your body is made up of 60 per cent water, which provides the fluid it needs to function efficiently both inside the cells and in the blood plasma and saliva. Many people do not drink enough water, and you can become dehydrated without even knowing it, especially when you exercise. The recommended intake is about six to eight glasses a day. When you exercise, make sure you sip water before, during and afterwards.

Vitamins and Minerals

Vitamins and minerals are essential for good health. Ideally, a balanced diet should provide all that the body needs, but even today with food in abundance in the western world there are vitamin deficiencies. These are normally caused by eating too much of a certain type of food and not enough of others. No single food will supply you with all the necessary vitamins and minerals – a healthy, balanced diet will.

losing **body fat**

Yฺou now understand the very basics of healthy eating, but if you are aiming to lose weight around your bum and tum you need to bear in mind the energy needs of your body. If the number of calories you take in is equal to the number you expend in everyday activities, then you are in energy balance; in other words, you won't put on any weight. If you take in more energy than the amount you expend, then you are likely to put on weight. If you take in less energy then you expend, your body will draw on stored energy and you will lose weight.

The aim here is not so much to lose weight as to lose excess body fat around your bum and tum. You can do this by following the tips for fat loss given below.

To Lose Body Fat
- Do not eat other people's leftovers
- Chew your food thoroughly
- Avoid eating fast food on the run
- Exercise regularly
- Only eat until you feel comfortable: better the excess in the bin than on your bum
- Eat foods that are low in fat
- Drink lots of water
- Eat complex carbohydrates and not simple sugars
- Eat moderate amounts of protein unless your doctor or a specialist has advised you otherwise (some people need more protein in their diet than others)
- Take a test at a health food store for any allergies or reactions to food

No More Crash Dieting
Hopefully, crash diets are today a thing of the past. We now know that our bodies respond to a drastic reduction of calories by lowering the metabolic rate to match our food intake and spare our energy stores. Your muscles respond to this in turn by reducing their mass and losing water.

Because your metabolism becomes so efficient during dieting, when you start to eat normally again your calorie needs will be less, so any extra intake of food after a period of restriction will become more than you need. The result will be that the excess is stored as body fat.

our bodies respond to a drastic reduction of calories by lowering the metabolic rate to match our food intake it's all in

your
mind

it's all in

Physical fitness has a beneficial effect on your mind as well as your body. Exercise has a positive effect on mood by creating a distraction from our stresses and strains and promoting **a sense of well-being**, which affects the way we feel about ourselves. The opposite is also true. Our mental outlook affects our physical body. Our thoughts and feelings are influenced by our senses. We take in information from the outside world, which we then represent on the inside through our **thoughts, feelings and experiences**. The language we use can bring about huge changes in our physiology and

your mind

our state of mind. For example, if you use negative language it is likely that you will have a negative outlook on life with emotions such as anxiety, worry or anger. This is likely to create tension on your physical body resulting in poor posture, aches and pains and health problems. A person who uses **positive language** is likely to have a more positive outlook, is less likely to carry tensions around with them and tends to have fewer health problems. We also need to explore how the mind can provide benefits for the physical body by directing our behaviour to become more motivated and focused.

We take in information from the world around us through our
sense organs. Everything we have ever seen, heard, felt,
smelt or tasted is taken in through the conscious part of our minds to
be stored in our subconscious forever! Most of us have one or two
senses that favour the others, and you can tell somebody's dominant
sensory system through the language they use and their physiology.
So have fun watching your friends.

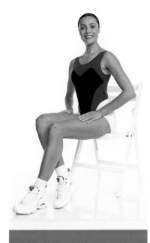

visual

If your language predominantly uses a lot of visual words like 'seeing
is believing' or 'looking good' or 'I see what you mean', then your
dominant sense would be visual. When we use visual language our
eyes will move upward or look straight ahead. A visual person is
most likely to be attracted to activities that are predominantly visual,
such as fashion, going to the movies or the visual arts. You may choose
a profession related to the arts and your motivational factor in exercise
is very likely to be to look good.

auditory

An auditory person will litter their conversation with sensory words like 'that party gave me a
great buzz' or 'this is music to my ears'. The eyes normally stay level and move left and right
or down and left. Your auditory system includes the making up and memories of sound. Exercise
to music might be a good motivational factor for you.

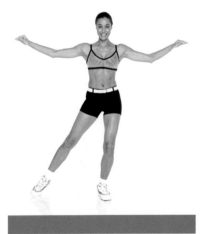

kinaesthetic

The kinaesthetic sensory system refers to feeling in both
an emotional and a tactile sense. If you use phrases
like 'I really feel that this is right for me' or 'She got right up
my nose!' and if you are quick to express your feelings
about things then you are likely to be a kinaesthetic
person. A kinaesthetic person is also likely to be more
sporty and have a greater sense of body awareness. You
may be naturally drawn to movement and choose active
professions such as physiotherapy, massage or fitness.

Which are you? I myself am mostly kinaesthetic, then
visual and pretty weak in the auditory department. I learn

best from hands-on experience and have had to work quite hard to develop my other senses. When you have worked out which is your dominant sense then you can use it for learning, or perhaps to explore the weaker senses and make them stronger. For example, the visual person who normally chooses to watch sport may want to translate her visual skills into action and consider different physical activities with which to explore her kinaesthetic sense. An auditory person could be motivated to explore fitness through reading about it or listening to tapes, and developing her visual sense through using her imagination or her kinaesthetic sense by choosing exercises that develop body awareness. A kinaesthetic person could develop her auditory skills by listening to music while she works, or she could read or write or explore visualisation to enhance her visual skills.

you can use your dominant sense for learning or to make weaker senses stronger

Each of these senses can be used as a powerful tool for learning and changing behaviour patterns to benefit you in every area of your life, but for the purposes of this book we are now going to explore these senses for body shaping.

55

visualisation

Visualisation is probably the most powerful natural tool you can develop. Research now shows that the brain does not differentiate between what is real and what is imaginary, so if you imagine yourself doing your exercises with good posture you will find that when it comes to exercising you will do so with good posture! If you have a positive outlook on life, this will show in your body, because the brain kick-starts the process of making these positive thoughts happen. Likewise, if you have a negative outlook it will show, and the brain will respond in the same way.

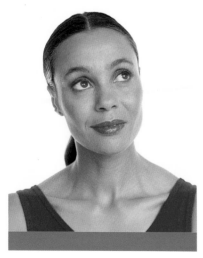

Studies have been carried out on people who were sedentary and had never exercised and on people who were also sedentary but visualised working their muscles with heavy weights. The result was that the people who visualised their muscles working had greater gains in strength. What the mind thinks, tends to happen! Visualisation is now considered to be an exceptionally valuable tool in sport, and world-class athletes are using mental image work to enhance their performances.

Visualisation is also considered valuable in disciplines such as neuro-linguistic programming and hypnotherapy.

Our visual sensory system makes all our mental pictures: the ones we remember and the ones we make up. When you visualise, you look up. For exercising your bum and tum you can start the process of positive thought by giving yourself the instruction to see yourself as you wish to be, with perfect posture, a flat tum and a toned bum. You can use visualisation to double-check your body alignment. It is, of course, essential to ensure that you visually remember the correct posture in the first place, so must check that you have taken in all the information you need to make sure that the picture you give yourself is correct.

affirmations

Verbalising something you want has a similar effect to visualisation, but this time by using the auditory part of the mind. Affirmations are positive statements that are repeated over and over again until the brain gets the message and starts to make changes to create a new habit or behavioural direction. The mind responds to the continual messages given to it, so if they are positive you will then respond in a positive way, but if you keep giving yourself negative statements then your behaviour is likely to become negative. When you use your auditory sense, your eyes look to either side to construct or to remember and down to the left for 'internal dialogue' or talking to yourself. For your 10-minute tone-ups, you can use your auditory skills to give yourself affirmations and encourage-ment to exercise properly. Talk yourself into good posture. Motivate yourself to achieve even more by telling yourself you can do a few more repetitions. You have the power within you to be your own personal trainer.

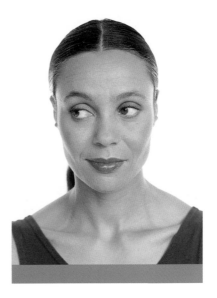

using your feelings

Last but by no means least, our feeling sense is a great human barometer! Often under-used, our feelings are a great indicator of what is going on in our lives – or not, as the case may be. If you can express your feelings you will probably find that you have a more positive outlook on life than someone who holds them in. Research also suggests that repressed feelings and emotions are contributory factors in medical conditions such as cancer, arthritis and depression, so being in tune with your feelings is essential. Kinaesthetic senses can be divided into two categories: those we experience as movement and those we experience from emotion. If you want to feel things more intensely, your eyes look down and to your right.

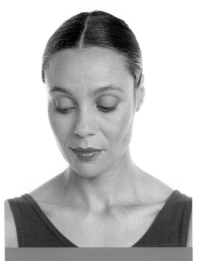

Studies have shown that when people are asked to pay close attention to how they feel in terms of exertion and fatigue, they are as accurate as scientific monitoring with heart-rate monitors and other equipment. So a really good way of assessing the intensity of your workout is to go by how you honestly feel. During exercise, use your imagination to conjure up a chart numbered from 1 to 10. Ask your mind to show you how hard you are working. Aim for about 6 to 7. In aerobic work, remember the talk test. At the end of exercise, look down and check how you are feeling. If you can hold a conversation easily then you are not working hard enough. If you can't hold one at all you are working too hard. Remember: you should just be comfortably out of breath.

putting it all **together**

Studies have shown that concentrating your mind on your muscles to create tension in them can give better control and extra resistance to a movement. This has the benefit of creating better technique and making your muscles work harder, which results in improved strength gains and tone in the muscles.

So, before you exercise, you need to spend a moment focusing on these sensory areas. You can do this by mentally visualising the areas that you are about to work as you want them to be – strong, toned and lean, with correct posture. You can use your verbal skills to talk yourself into position.

Lastly, you can use your kinaesthetic senses to become conscious of how and what you should feel and also how to focus your mind on your muscle to push yourself a little harder.

visualisation for
a perfect tum and bum

The following relaxation exercise will help you with these skills. I would suggest that you start practising your auditory skills by reading the instructions into a tape and then playing it when you have a moment to relax.

This exercise will also start to direct changes in your mind towards your goal of the perfect tum and bum.

● Begin by taking a few deep breaths, inhaling through your nose and exhaling through your mouth. As you breathe, make sure that you are using the whole of your lungs to fill every nerve, muscle and cell in your body with life-giving oxygen. Feel your ribs lifting as you breathe in and falling as you breathe out.

● Turn your attention to all the muscles in your body, tensing and tightening each and every one, and then releasing so that they are completely relaxed. Start from your feet and work your way up through your calves, thighs, buttocks, trunk, chest, back, shoulders, arms, neck and head.

● Now allow waves of relaxation to flow throughout your body until every nerve, muscle and cell is completely relaxed. As you become more and more relaxed, be aware of the rhythm of your breath moving in and out, in and out. Focus on this natural rhythm and spend a few moments clearing your mind of all clutter as you breathe.

● Imagine that you are in a movie house, sitting about halfway between front and back. As you seat yourself comfortably, an image of you as you are fills the screen. Explore that image. Really take a good look at your body, your posture and your shape, particularly around your tum and bum. Acknowledge all the good things about yourself and be aware of your natural body shape. Now focus on the areas that you want to improve, your tum and bum, and know that you have the resources inside you right now to make those changes. Be aware of those resources, and put them up on the screen now.

acknowledge all the good things about yourself and be aware of your natural body shape

● See yourself doing the things that you need to do to make those changes possible. See yourself now exercising regularly, focusing on the two different areas of your body – your abdominal and buttock muscles. Feel your muscles developing as you exercise, becoming tighter, more toned and stronger;

58

tighter, more toned and stronger. Hear your voice repeating, 'My muscles are becoming tighter, more toned and stronger every time I exercise.'

● See yourself putting more energy into your daily activities and be aware of what that feels like. Hear the compliments that others are giving you as changes are beginning to be noticed. More importantly, hear the compliments that you give yourself, and be aware of the sense of achievement, confidence and well-being that you feel as a result of the effort you are putting in.

see yourself putting more energy into your daily activities

● Now be aware of your new eating habits: low-fat food, lots of fruit and vegetables, and plenty of water to drink. See yourself looking more closely at the nutritional value on the back of food packs. Be aware of your voice telling you when you are comfortably full and that there is no need to eat any more. See yourself going through the process of sorting out old clothes in your wardrobe, trying them on and delighting when you know that they now fit you. See the delight in your face, feel the delight in your body and hear the delight in your voice.

● As you go through all these resources in your mind, take another look at the screen more closely now. You begin to be aware of the changes in your body. You are looking leaner and more toned, and your posture is improving in every way. Hold this image of the new you firmly in your mind and explore it.

● Now imagine yourself getting up from your seat and walking towards the movie screen. Take one last look and make any changes you want to the image on the screen, then step into the image and be that new you: fitter, more toned and confident, with a flat tum and a tight, toned bum.

● Explore what it feels like to be the new you, and what it looks like to have this new shape. Know that you can draw upon this image any time, any place you like. Now let the image fade away. Before you either drift off to sleep or come out of relaxation, imagine what you will look like in three months' time after all the hard work you will have put in, and then in six months' time. See what you see, hear what you hear and feel what you feel. When you are ready, either drift off to sleep or become wide awake.

The objective of this last section is to 'pace' the outcome of this exercise for the future. You will know that if you have a positive outcome then the exercise you have just done will make a lasting impression by creating positive changes in your mind. If you do not have a positive image of how you want to be, then further work needs to be done through more visualisation. Practise until you are aware of sensing a more positive image.

59

post

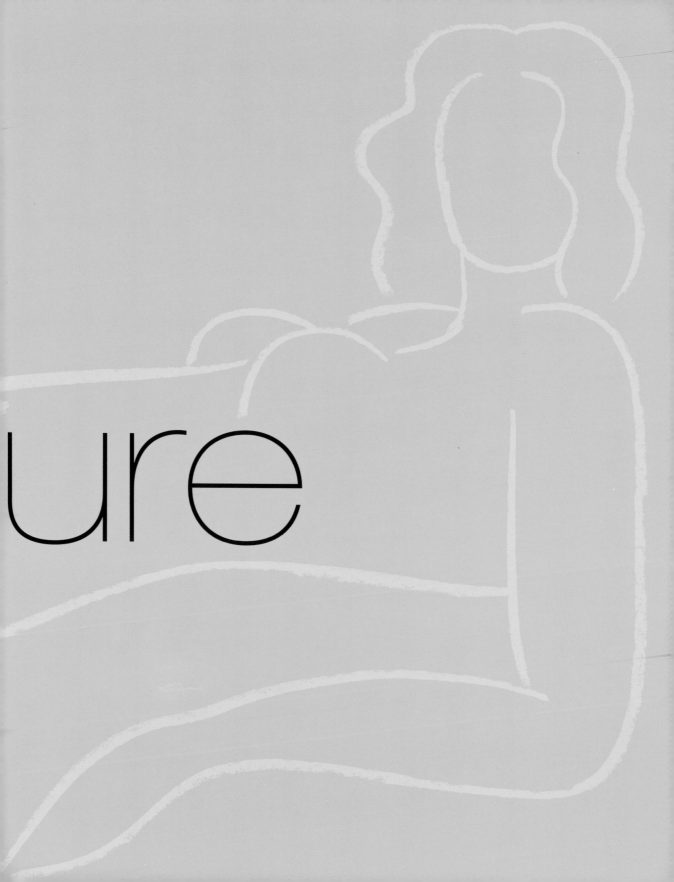

ure

posture

Before embarking on any exercise regime, and particularly if performing exercises involving postural muscles, such as the abdominal and buttock muscles, you need to **look at your body alignment**. The way you hold yourself influences the way you look and feel. It can also have a marked effect on the shape and condition of your body, creating shortness and tightness in some muscles and over-lengthening and weakness in others. Your posture is the **foundation for good stability** from which you can move, and like any foundation that becomes unstable, poor body alignment will have a knock-on effect on the rest of your body.

Before you start toning your muscles, you need to look at the **relationship between the muscle groups** and the effect that they have on the body when compromised. Your aim is to **redress the imbalance** in those groups by spending 10 minutes a day getting them into alignment before you move on to the stronger work later in the book.

Body alignment is an intrinsic part of an exercise programme and one that is frequently ignored. Too often we think we can skip the basics because they seem so easy and move on to the next level to be more challenged. But many people, especially in the sports industry, are discovering that missing out the basics has a detrimental effect on their bodies, creating structural imbalance, which can end up as injuries. Good body alignment influences your shape and the way you feel about yourself, so I would strongly urge you to pay special attention to this chapter before moving on.

your buttock muscles

Research now shows that well-toned and flexible buttock muscles play a central role in posture, affecting the stability of your hips, the positioning of your pelvis and the balance of the musculature around these areas. Your spine is the focal point from which the upper and lower body work. If the hips are not well balanced, then both upper and lower body can be affected, particularly the back and the knees. Say, for example, that your main buttock muscle is slack, it is then likely that the opposite muscle group, the hip flexors, will be short and tight, and this in turn has an effect on the positioning of your pelvis, creating an exaggerated inward curve of your lower back.

the golden rule is to include movements to promote stability of the hips and back

Your buttock muscles also play a role in dynamic posture, that is your posture when you move. When you walk, you place your weight through your foot. Your gluteus medius and gluteus minimus muscles contract to ensure that the hip is stable throughout the movement. If your hips are not stable, then when you walk you are likely to develop a rolling gait. Other movements, such as climbing the stairs, can also be affected.

The golden rule in any exercise regime is to include movements that will promote the stability of the hips and back to help achieve good posture around the pelvic area. Before you do the bum exercises in Chapters 8 to 10, make sure you spend some time working on the alignment of your buttock muscles with the exercises in this chapter.

If you are having treatment for any postural faults, check with your chartered physiotherapist before performing these exercises.

your **hip flexors**

In opposition to the buttock muscles are the hip flexors, which are at the top of the front of your thigh. These are the muscles that bring your knees towards your chest. If you have a job where you are sitting all day then you could have hip flexors that are tight, especially if you are not doing any walking or other exercise. However, these muscles can also be excessively lengthened. Your hip flexors play an important role in balancing the muscles of the hip and should always be stretched whenever you have worked your buttock muscles.

your **abdominal muscles**

We saw in Chapter 2 that the spine is like a series of building blocks, with one vertebra stacked on top of another. Poor posture can change the dynamics of the spine, placing it out of alignment and making it unstable and open to injury.

The abdominal muscles play a major role in keeping the body in alignment by acting as a stabiliser to the lower back, but even they can easily be affected by lifestyle. For example, excess weight and inactivity can leave your abdominals weak and poorly toned. Having a baby can also stretch and weaken them, as can any form of abdominal surgery. Wearing high heels will affect the tilt of your pelvis and cause an increased curvature of your spine, and this has the effect of over-lengthening the abdominals.

The muscles that play the most important role in posture are the transverse abdominal muscles, which are responsible for the stability of the spine. If your transverse muscles are weak then your back is more vulnerable; when they are well conditioned you have a stronger centre from which to work. In exercise, there is a tendency to ignore the transverse abdominals and concentrate on doing lots of sit-ups. The result is that the muscles responsible for movement become strong but the deeper stability muscles remain weak.

The aim here is to spend 10 minutes a day redressing the balance in muscle tone that can create an uneven pull on your bum and tum. You can do this by using stretching exercises to lengthen tight muscles, combined with strengthening exercises to tighten and tone slack muscles.

posture test

Stand up against a wall with your feet slightly apart and about 9–10 cm (3–4 in) away from it. Make sure your bum and shoulder muscles are relaxed and touching the wall (1). Place your hand between the wall and the lower part of your back (2). If the whole of your hand goes through, then it is likely that your pelvis tilts too far forward and your lower back is too arched. If you can't get your fingers through at all, then it is likely that your pelvis tilts too far back and your back is too flat. The ideal posture is when you can place your fingers through the gap.

Go to a mirror and look at what you have discovered at the wall. You now know that your pelvis is in either the wrong or the right position and that the alignment of your lower back is influenced by that position.

Spend a moment now side-on, with your feet shoulder width apart, your knees slightly soft and your upper body relaxed. Gently tilt your pelvis forwards and backwards and then from side to side. The ideal posture is when your pelvis is tilted neither too far forward nor too far back. It needs to be in a neutral position with a natural curve in your lower back.

No matter how fit you are, I would strongly urge you to perform the following exercises before moving on to the workouts later in the book.

you now know if your pelvis is in the wrong or right position

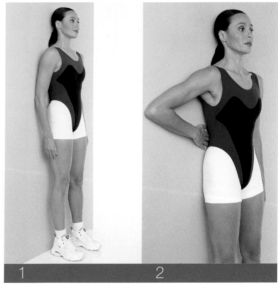

1   2

The following exercises redress the balance of a hollow back posture. But everybody should exercise their abdominal and buttock muscles to ensure strength and stability of the spine.

redressing **the balance**

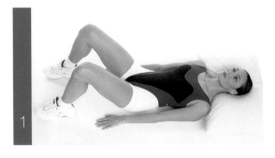

◀ tummy tightener

1 You may want to place a cushion under your head for comfort. Lie on your back with your knees bent and feet slightly apart. Starting in the groin area, begin to draw in the lower part of your abdominals and flatten your back to the floor.

2 Hold for 2 counts and then release for 4 counts. Build up to holding (and releasing) for 5 counts.

you should feel a pulling sensation in your lower tummy; make sure your back stays flat

▶ waist tightener

Lie on your back as for the tummy tightener and draw in your lower abdominals as before. While holding the contraction, bring your opposite hand and knee together and push them slightly against each other. Hold for 2 counts and then release for 4 counts. Repeat on the other side. Build up the hold to 8 to 10 counts.

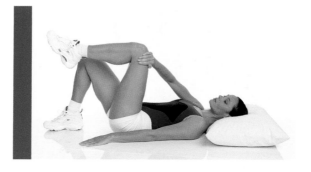

make sure your upper body remains relaxed and your back flat; do not hold your breath

▶ buttock tightener

Whenever you do any buttock exercises you need to contract your abdominals consciously. This will make the buttock muscles work more effectively. Lie face down with your hips on a cushion. Keep your legs straight. Hold in your abdominals and squeeze your buttocks. Now lift one foot about 8 cm (3 in) off the floor and take your leg out to the side by 15–20 cm (6–8 in), squeezing your buttocks as you do so. Hold for 2 counts and then slowly come back to the centre for 2 counts. Repeat with the other leg.

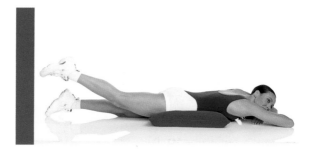

make sure your hips are pressed to the floor throughout

▶ back toner

Lie on the floor on your tummy with your feet slightly apart. Your hands can be on your bum or on the floor, with palms up. Keeping your hips pressed to the floor, use your lower back muscles to lift your shoulders off the ground for 2 counts, then lower for 2 counts.

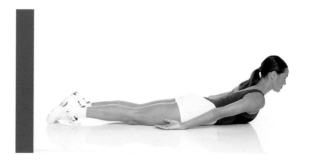

It is essential to make sure you stretch your muscles. When you tone them, they can become tighter and more inflexible. Stretching reduces muscular tension and keeps muscles more supple.

stretches

▶ front thigh and hip flexor stretch

Find a chair or table that is about 15 cm (6 in) higher than your knee. Stand with your feet slightly apart and in an upright position, with your abdominals held in. Bend your supporting leg so that your knee is slightly soft. Bring the other foot up behind you and use your toes to hook your foot on to the chair. Tilt your pelvis under to prevent you from arching your back. Hold this stretch for between 10 and 30 seconds. Repeat with the other leg.

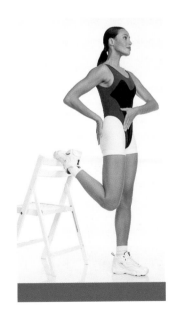

make sure your knee faces the floor and your abdominals are held in tight

▶ back stretch 1

Lie on your back, then hug your knees towards your chest with your hands behind them. Hold for between 10 and 30 seconds.

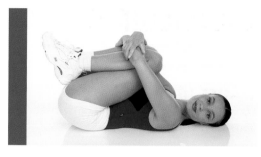

keep your body relaxed; breathe normally

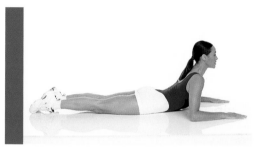

◀ back stretch 2

Lie on your front with your elbows bent and hands flat on the floor. Gently lift your head and shoulders off the floor by pushing on your hands until you feel a stretch down your tummy. Hold for between 10 and 30 seconds.

If you find you have strain in your back or that it is over-arching, lower your elbows to the floor or omit this exercise

look straight ahead of you and think about lengthening your spine; keep your hips on the floor; make sure you find a level that is comfortable

▶ buttock stretch

Lie on your back, then bend your right knee towards you and place your left foot on the floor with the knee bent. Take your right foot across your left knee. Now bring your left knee up towards you with your hands at the back of the knee, and hold for between 10 and 30 seconds. Repeat with the other leg.

If you find this exercise difficult, try to keep your left foot flat on the floor and your right foot across your left knee. Sit up with your hands on the floor behind you for support.

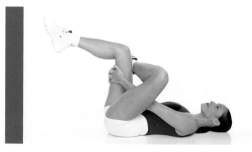

relax your upper body and make sure you keep your back straight

posture workout

WARM-UP

Spend about 30 seconds on each of these warm-up exercises from Chapter 7.

- **waist twists**
- **hip rolls**
- **spinal bridge**
- **march on the spot**

TONING

Spend about 30 seconds on each exercise (or each side, where these are worked separately).

- **tummy tightener**
- **buttock tightener**
- **waist tightener**
- **back toner**

71

STRETCHES

Hold each stretch for between 10 and 30 seconds.

- **hip flexor stretch**
  as you progress, use the stretches in Chapters 8, 9 and 10
- **back stretch 1**
- **buttock stretch**
- **back stretch 2**

Work at your own pace. Initially, 2 sets of the toning exercises may be too much and you will find yourself going over 10 minutes, but as you get used to the movements they will come with ease. Take your time getting into position.

warming

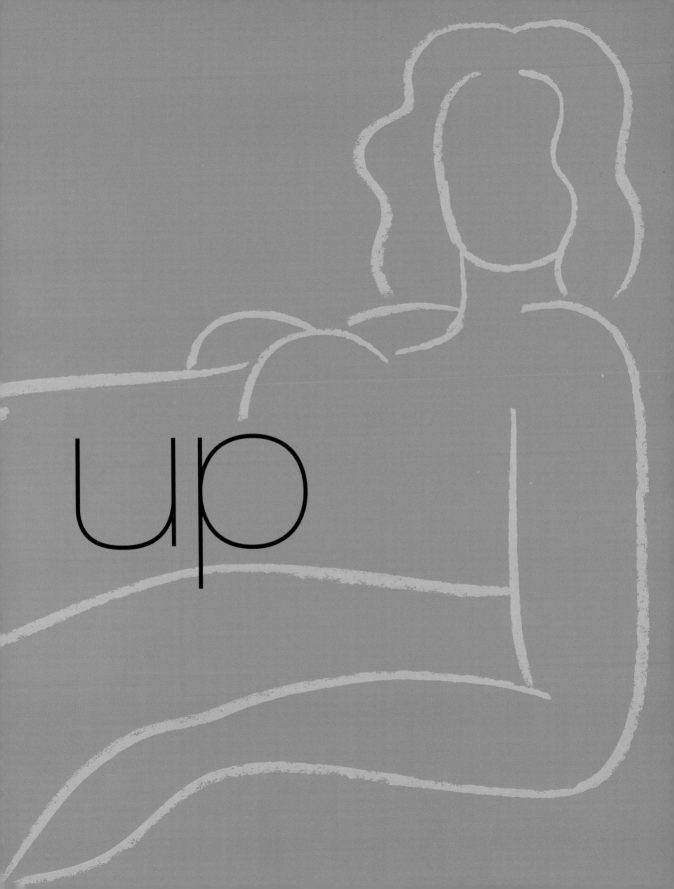

warming up

Before you begin toning your tum and bum **you need to warm up**. When the body is cold, joints and muscles are stiff and less pliable, and can be damaged more easily. A few minutes' preparation before starting to exercise is most beneficial. You can also prepare for physical activity by making sure you are in **a relaxed frame of mind**: the more relaxed and focused you are, the more likely you are to enjoy and make the most of your exercises. You can achieve this by spending a moment or two concentrating on your breath.

breathing

Breathing properly is important, as breathing high in the chest shows tension and uses only the top part of the lungs. You want to make sure that you breathe lower down in the chest, enabling your chest and ribs to expand more fully. Another common habit is to hold the breath; this not only restricts the amount of oxygen entering your body but can also raise your blood pressure, which is not beneficial for health.

Start by kneeling in a comfortable position with your shoulders relaxed. Now spend a moment regulating your breathing. As you breathe, place a hand over your diaphragm and feel the rise and fall of your chest. Now visualise it: it should be the lower part of your ribs and the triangular area between the curve of your lower ribs that rises and falls gently.

You must also make sure that you use your breath properly during exercise. The general rule is to breathe out with effort, which means you breathe in just before a movement takes place, and exhale during the effort of the movement.

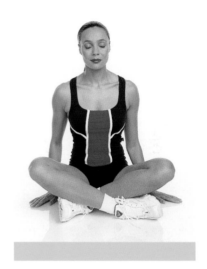

75

warming up

When warming up muscles and joints it is essential to do it gradually. As you warm up, deep muscle temperature is raised and joints become looser as fluid is released. This has the effect of making ligaments, tendons and muscle fibres more pliable, increasing the range of movement of the joint as well as protecting your body from injury.

As the muscles you are working are those of your bum and tum, the area to focus on loosening up is the spine, the pelvis – which is connected to the lumbar spine – and the hip joints. However, if you are working one muscle group daily then just do the necessary mobility and warm-up exercises for that area. For example, if you are working on your tum, do the pelvic tilt, spinal bridge and waist twists. You may also want to march on the spot to increase your body temperature. If you are working your bum, do the pelvic tilt, hip rolls, knee raises and the toe-tapping exercises to the side and behind. Do each exercise until you feel loose and warm. It is ideal to stretch the muscle groups you are working both before and after exercise. Hold warm-up stretches for 8 to 10 seconds and cool-down stretches for 15 to 30 seconds to develop flexibility. Do each exercise until you feel loose and warm.

It is ideal to stretch the muscle groups you are working with both before and after exercise. Before starting the warm-up, remember your exercise posture (see Chapter 6). The first exercise, the pelvic tilt, should be practised throughout the day, not just when exercising. Spend a moment visualising the spine in its neutral position and tell yourself that your spine will be in this alignment at all times.

tum **warm up**

▶ **pelvic tilt**

Stand with your feet shoulder width apart, knees slightly soft and upper body relaxed. Tighten your abdominal muscles. Gently tilt your pelvis backwards and forwards, and then find the neutral position between the two.

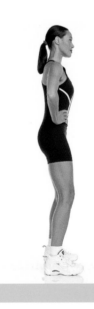

make sure your abdominals remain tight; check that your movements are controlled; maintain a lengthened posture

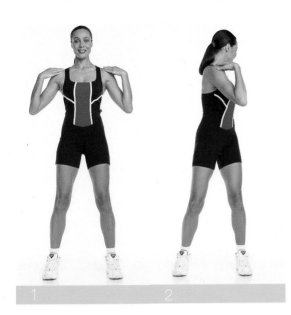

◀ **waist twists**

1 Stand with your feet shoulder width apart, knees slightly bent and a neutral spine. Tighten your abdominals and keep your hips perfectly still and facing forwards.

2 Gently twist your shoulders and head to the right, then return to the centre and twist to the left.

make sure your abdominals are held in; check that your hips are facing forwards

▶ **spinal bridge**

1 Stand with your feet shoulder width apart, your knees bent, and leaning forwards, with your hands on your thighs for support.

2 Keep your abdominals tight and spine neutral. Lift up through your spine like a cat to round your back, and then gently release to the neutral spine position.

relax your shoulders; do not over-arch your back

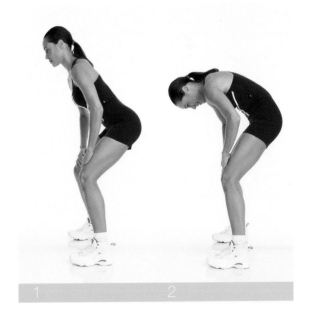

Now march on the spot until you feel warm.

bum warm up

▶ **pelvic tilt**

Stand with your feet shoulder width apart, knees slightly soft and upper body relaxed. Tighten your abdominals. Gently tilt your pelvis backwards and forwards and then find the neutral position. Now do the same from side to side.

make sure that your abdominals are held in tight; check that your shoulders are relaxed and gently held down

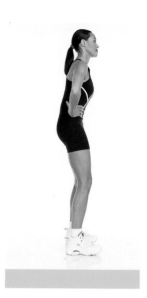

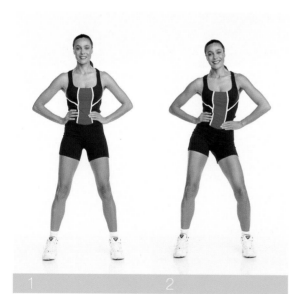

1   2

◀ **hip rolls**

1 Stand with your feet shoulder width apart, knees slightly soft and upper body relaxed. Tighten your abdominals.

2 Now start gently rocking your pelvis backwards and forwards and from side to side, until the movement becomes a circle. Do 8 to 10 circles each way. Use smooth controlled movements

make sure your body remains centred as you circle

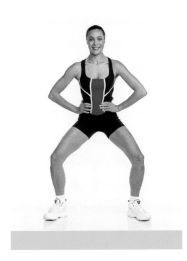

◀ knee bends

Stand with your feet shoulder width apart, hands on hips and your toes turned out slightly. Hold your abdominals in and keep your upper body relaxed. Bend your knees and then straighten. Do 8 to 10 repetitions.

check that your knees are in line with your toes and not going beyond them

▶ side tap

Stand with your feet together and hands on hips. Hold your abdominals in. Tap your right leg out to the side bringing your arms out to the side at the same time, bring it back to the centre and then change legs. Alternate between the two until your body starts to feel warm.

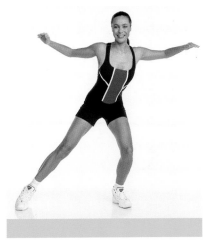

keep your supporting leg soft as you tap the other one to the side; hold in your abdominals

▶ tap behind

Stand with your feet slightly apart and abdominals held in. Place your hands on your hips and lean forward slightly. Tap your right foot behind you, bring it back to the starting position and then tap your left foot behind you. Squeeze your buttock muscles as you move. Do 20 repetitions, or as many as you need to start feeling warm.

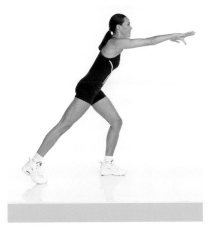

Now march on the spot until you feel warm.

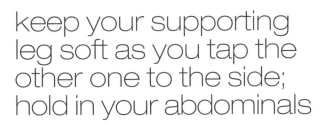

beginner's

work
out

beginner's

The workouts in this chapter have been designed to be **achievable and effective in a short space of time**, and to make sure that you have a well-balanced exercise programme. While you are focusing primarily on your tum and bum, it is also important to **consider the other muscle groups** around the area in order to avoid muscular imbalance.

You may find that when you are first learning how to do these exercises you do not have time to do all of them and your stretches. That's fine. Just

workout

focus on getting the quality right before moving on to the next exercise. When I have limited time, I focus on one muscle group and really make sure that I have overloaded it. I then **stretch the muscles** I have just worked. On the next day, I choose another muscle group, and so on. What is important is balance, so if you only have time to do a buttock squeeze and a sit-down squat, for example, make sure you stretch the hip flexors and other muscle groups worked, not a totally different muscle group.

For this exercise programme you are limited to 10 minutes, so you will generally be working on one set of each exercise. Do not hurry these exercises. It is better to do less and be sure of quality movement.

tum exercises

▶ lying pelvic tilt

1 Lie on the floor with your feet apart and knees bent, upper body relaxed and hands by your sides. Tighten your abdominal and buttock muscles and tilt your pelvis up and then back.

2 Now repeat the movement and stop at the midpoint between the two so that your spine is in a neutral position. Pull your abdominals in tight and hold for 4 counts, then release for 4 counts. Build up to 15 to 20 repetitions.

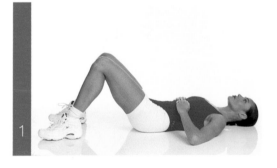

1

do not hold your breath; use smooth, controlled movements

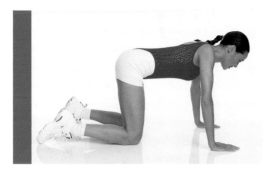

◀ tummy tightener

Kneel on all fours with your knees under your hips and hands directly under your shoulders. Your head should be in line with the rest of your body. Let your abdominals relax completely, then draw them up and in tight from your pubic bone to your navel. Hold for 30 seconds, building up to 1 minute. Keep your spine still and flat like the top of a table.

▶ basic curl-up

1 Lie on your back with your knees bent and feet flat on the floor. Tilt your pelvis to neutral and tighten your abdominals.

2 Use your tummy muscles to lift your shoulders off the floor, reaching forwards with your fingers towards your heels. Hold for 2 counts, then lower for 4 counts. Build up to 15 to 20 repetitions.

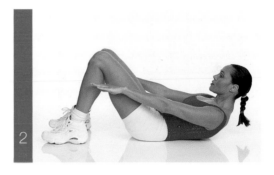

85

relax your head and neck; breathe out with the effort and do not hold your breath; squeeze your abdominals in tight throughout

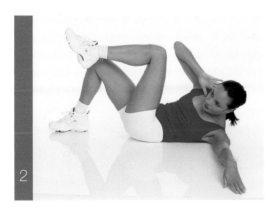

◀ waist tightener

1 Lie with your feet apart and flat on the floor, with your knees bent. Place one hand behind your ear with your elbow bent and the other hand out on the floor for support.

2 Tighten your abdominals and curl up and over diagonally for 2 counts by bringing your shoulder towards the opposite knee. Lower for 2 counts. Do 15 to 20 repetitions on each side.

tum stretches

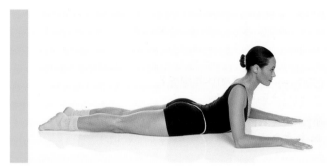

◀ abdominal stretch

Lie on your tummy and place your hands on the floor in front of you at shoulder level, so that your elbows are in line with your shoulders. Push up on to your elbows by lifting your head and shoulders off the floor. Hold for 15 seconds, building up to 30 seconds.

keep your hips, elbows and feet on the floor

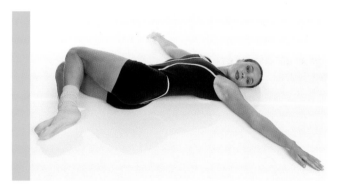

◀ waist stretch

Lie on your back with your knees bent and arms out at shoulder level. Let your knees drop over to one side and hold for 15 seconds before changing to the other side. Build up to holding for 30 seconds.

keep your feet together and both shoulders on the floor; breathe normally throughout

beginner's
tum workout

WARM-UP

Spend about 30 seconds on these mobility exercises from Chapter 7, along with a 1-minute march and 15-second full body stretch.

- **waist twists**
- **march on the spot**
- **spinal bridge**
- **full body stretch** (see page 101)

TONING

Spend about 30 seconds on each exercise (or each side, where these are worked separately).

87

- **lying pelvic tilt**
- **basic curl-up**
- **tummy tightener**
- **waist tightener**

STRETCHES

Hold each stretch for 15 to 30 seconds.

- **abdominal stretch**
- **full body stretch** (see page 101)
- **waist stretch**

Make sure you allow yourself time to get into each position. When you are able to go from one position to the next with ease, you may use the time to increase the number of repetitions or to stretch and relax.

This section focuses primarily on your buttock muscles. The aim is to keep the spine protected at all times, so think about keeping your back as flat as possible and your abdominals held in.

bum exercises

▶ buttock squeeze

1 Lie on your back, tighten your abdominals and tilt your pelvis as you would in a pelvic tilt. Keep your hands down by your sides.

2 Keeping your abdominals tight, lift your hips off the floor slightly and squeeze your buttocks for 2 counts, then gently release for 2 counts. Build up to 20 repetitions.

keep your hips
still and do not
over-arch
your back

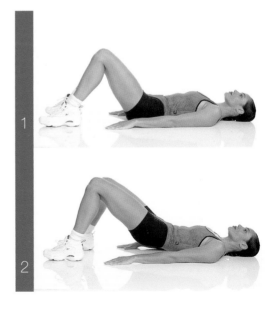

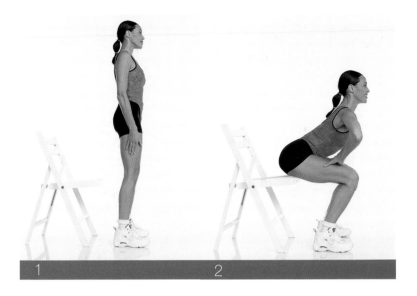

▲ sit-down squat

1 Stand in front of a chair (with a seat no lower than your knee line) with your feet shoulder width apart and toes facing forwards. Place your hands on your thighs.

2 Lean forwards, pulling your abdominals in, and press your hips out behind you as if to sit in the chair for 2 counts. Allow your buttocks to touch the seat of the chair before pushing through your heels and standing up again for 4 counts. Build up to 15 to 20 repetitions.

keep your back flat and look straight ahead

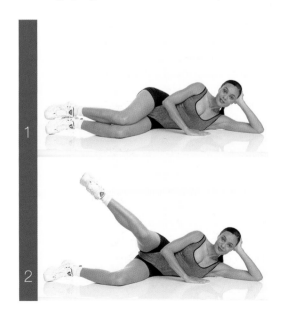

◀ outer thigh raise

1 Lie on your side with your thighs together, one on top of the other. Rest your head on your hand. Bring both knees forwards about 45 degrees.

2 then rotate the top knee by about 2.5 cm (1 in) so that the knee is facing inwards towards the floor and the heel is facing the ceiling. Keeping your hips forwards, raise the top leg for 2 counts and lower for 2 counts, squeezing your buttocks as you move your leg. Build up to 15 to 20 repetitions. Repeat on the other side.

your hips should remain still and your top knee dip in

▶ inner thigh raise

1 Lie on your side with one leg on top of the other. Rest your head on your hand. Bring your top leg in front of you, resting your knee on a cushion.

2 Lift your underneath leg for 2 counts and lower for 2 counts. Build up 15 to 20 repetitions. Repeat on the other side.

make sure your
foot faces forwards;
check that your
hips face forwards

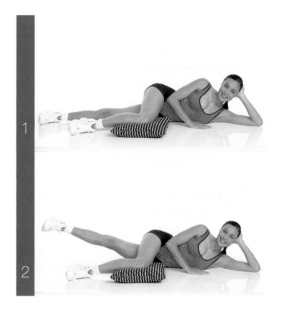

bum stretches

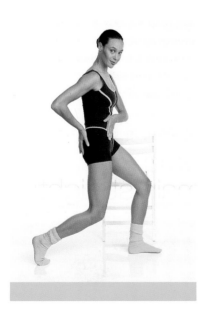

◀ hip flexor stretch

You may need a wall or chair to help you with balance. Stand with your feet together. Take one leg behind you, lifting the heel off the ground. Bend your knees by about 15 cm (6 in), tuck your pelvis under and hold this position for 15 seconds. Repeat with the other leg.

make sure your feet
are facing forwards;
keep your abdominals
in tight; check that your
upper body is upright

▶ front thigh stretch

You may need a wall or chair for support. Stand with your feet together. Shift your weight on to one leg and soften the knee. Bring the heel of the opposite leg up towards your buttocks and reach for the ankle. Tighten your abdominals and hold on to the ankle, tuck your pelvis under and make sure your knee faces the floor. Hold the stretch for 15 seconds. Repeat with the other leg.

make sure you hold your abdominals in; your back should remain flat and your thighs parallel

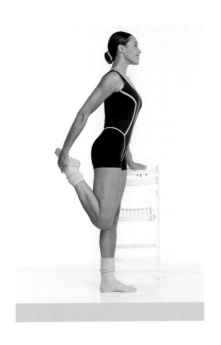

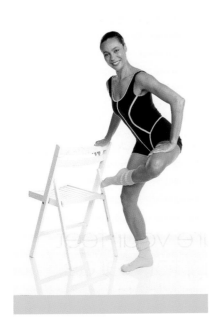

◀ buttock stretch

Stand about 30 cm (12 in) away from a wall or chair and hold it for support, then bend your supporting leg slightly. Bring the ankle of the opposite leg up and across the knee of the supporting leg, so that it looks as if you are crossing your legs standing up. Keeping your ankle over your knee, pull your abdominals in and bend the knee of your supporting leg. Allow your upper body to lean forwards. Hold for 15 seconds. Repeat with the other leg.

your hips should stay centred and your back remain straight; keep your head in line with your body

▶ hamstring stretch

Start with your feet together. Extend one leg forwards and bend the other slightly. Placing your hands on the tops of your thighs, tighten your abdominals and lean your body forwards from the hips. Hold for 15 seconds. Repeat with the other leg. Make sure your head is in line with your body.

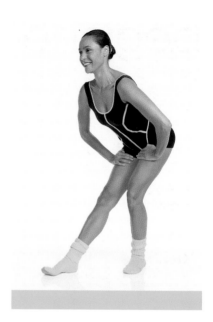

keep your chest lifted and your back straight; press your hips further behind you to increase the stretch

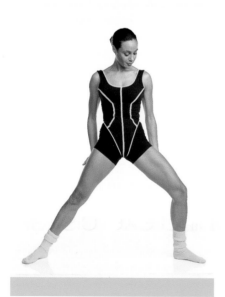

◀ inner thigh stretch

Stand with your feet wider than shoulder width apart and turned out slightly, keeping your body in an upright position. Keep your hips facing forwards and your chest lifted. Bend one leg while keeping the other leg straight. The foot of your straight leg should remain flat on the floor. Place your hands on your thighs for support and lean forwards slightly so that you are leaning into the stretch. Hold for 15 seconds. Repeat with the other leg.

make sure your knees are in line with your toes – you may have to adjust your foot position

beginner's
bum workout

WARM UP

Spend about 30 seconds on these mobility exercises from Chapter 7.

- **hip rolls**
- **side tap**
- **knee bends**
- **tap behind**

TONING

Spend about 30 seconds on each exercise (or each side, where these are worked separately).

- **buttock squeeze**
- **outer thigh raise**
- **sit-down squat**
- **inner thigh raise**

93

STRETCHES

Hold each stretch for 15 seconds.

- **front thigh stretch**
- **buttock stretch or wall knee raise**
- **hamstring stretch**
- **inner thigh stretch**

When you first start you may only have time to do 1 set of the toning exercises, but you will soon progress to 2 sets. The more familiar the exercises become, the quicker you'll be able to get into position. Technique is of the utmost importance.

intermediate

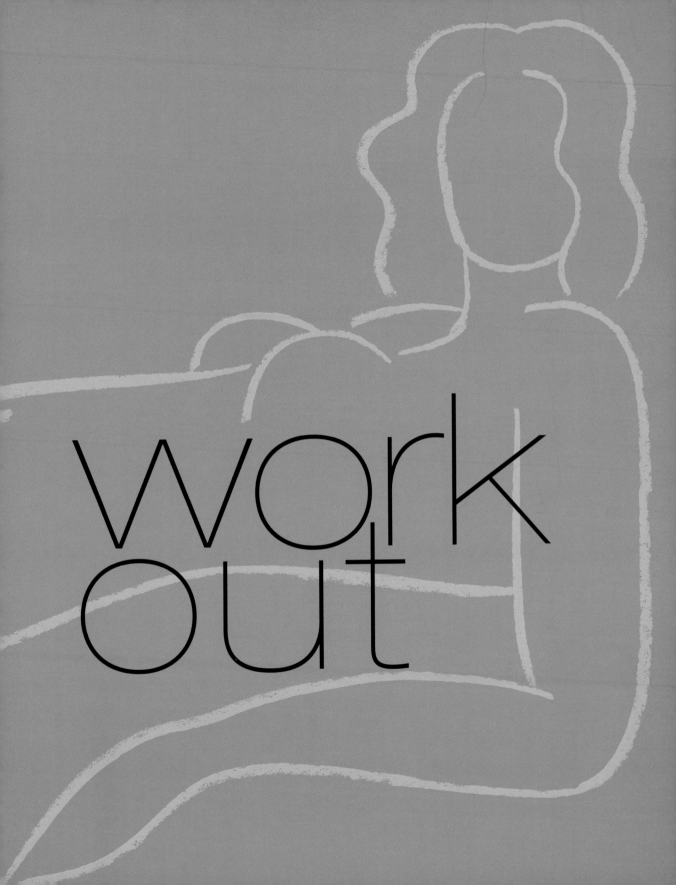

work
out

intermediate

Once your fitness levels have improved to the point where the exercises in Chapter 8 are no longer as challenging as when you first started them, you are ready to move on to the next stage. In order to progress, you need to **stimulate your muscles** some more, and the exercises in this chapter achieve this by changing the level of leverage and resistance, thereby **increasing the intensity**. Remember: these exercises are

workout

different from the others. When you are trying out new exercises take your time and allow yourself time to adjust to the new movement. Be aware of what the new movement looks like and what it feels like. **Use your auditory skills** to coach your body into position. Success comes when you focus on what you are doing, and then make sure that you perform each exercise perfectly. Above all, **practise, practise, practise!**

The following abdominal exercises will be more challenging. Work at your own pace, get into the right position and use your visualisation skills to enhance your performance.

tum exercises

▶ tummy tightener

1 Begin by kneeling on all fours, with your hands shoulder width apart and directly under your shoulders. Now go down on to your elbows and lean forward with your hips.

2 Adjust your elbows so that they are directly under your shoulders and keep your back flat. Hold your abdominals in tight. Build up the hold to between 45 seconds and 1 minute.

do not stick your bottom up or hold your breath

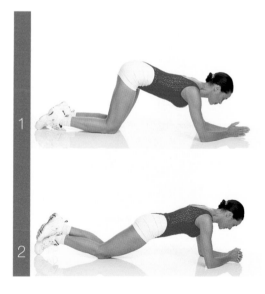

▸ hands-crossed curl-up

1 Lie on your back with your feet slightly apart and knees bent, and your spine in the neutral position. Cross your hands over your chest.

2 Tighten your abdominals and use them to lift your head and shoulders off the ground for 2 counts, then lower for 4 counts. Breathe out as you come up and in as you lower. Build up to 15 to 20 repetitions.

do not strain your neck; tighten your abdominals as you curl up

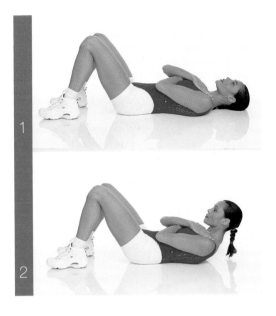

99

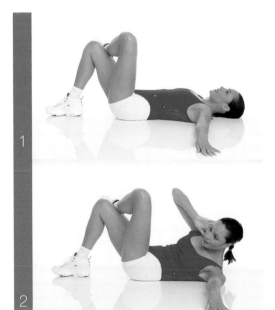

◂ waist tightener

1 Lie on your back with your feet slightly apart. Bring your left ankle across your right knee and your left arm out to the side for support. Place your right hand behind your right ear.

2 Tighten your abdominals and bring your right shoulder towards your left knee for 2 counts and then back for 2 counts. Build up to 15 to 20 repetitions on each side.

make sure your hips are firmly on the floor; do not pull on your head

▶ reverse curl

1 Lie on your back with your hands down by your sides. Bend your knees so that your feet are off the floor and your knees are over your hips at about 90 degrees. Tighten your abdominals.

2 Gently tilt your pelvis up towards the ceiling by bringing your knees towards your chest for 2 counts, then lower for 2 counts. Build up to 15 to 20 repetitions.

do not swing your legs or rock; relax your arms, neck and shoulders; lower smoothly

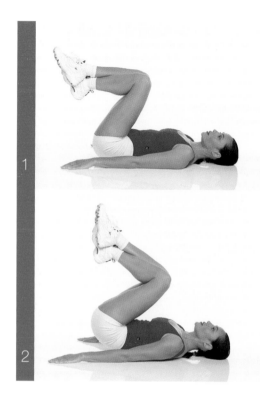

At all times during exercise you need to breathe evenly, making sure that your breaths are rhythmical and natural. You should breathe out with every effort that you make.

tum **stretches**

▶ **full body stretch**

Lie on your back with your hands by your sides. Bring your arms above your head and stretch them in both directions as far as you can. Hold the stretch for 15 seconds, building up to 30 seconds over time.

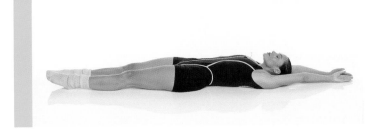

do not over-arch your back; do not hold your breath

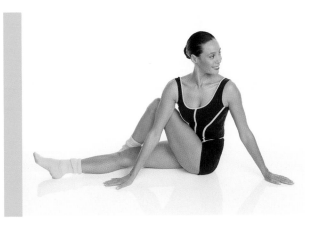

◀ **waist stretch**

Sit with your legs straight out in front of you. Now bend your left leg, crossing your left foot to rest over your right knee. Bring your right elbow over to the outside of your left knee. Make sure your left hand is on the ground for support. Gently turn your head to look over your left shoulder and gently rotate your upper body to the left. Hold this position for 15 seconds. Repeat on the other side.

keep your hips still and both buttocks on the floor; do not use jerky movements or bounce

intermediate
tum workout

WARM UP

As for the beginner's workout.

TONING

Spend up to 1 minute on the tummy tightener, and about 30 seconds on each of the other exercises (or on each side, where these are worked separately).

- **tummy tightener**
- **waist tightener**
- **hands-crossed curl-up**
- **reverse curl**

STRETCHES

Hold each stretch for 15 to 30 seconds.

- **abdominal stretch** (see page 86)
- **waist stretch**
- **full body stretch**

Transitions between exercises and positions should be easier now. Perform each exercise more slowly and hold the stretches for longer.

By now you will be familiar with working your buttock muscles, so you should cope well with the following exercises. Work your muscles smoothly through their full range of movement.

bum exercises

▸ **one-legged buttock squeeze**
Lie on your back, tighten your abdominals and do a pelvic tilt. Keep your hands by your sides. Bring your right foot over your left knee and place it on your left thigh. Tighten both your buttock muscles and lift your hips off the floor. Squeeze your left buttock for 2 counts and release for 2 counts. Repeat with the other leg.

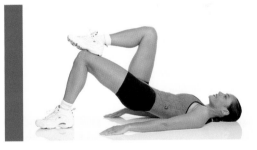

keep your hips still and your abdominals held in tight; do not over-arch your back; do not hold your breath

▶ wide squat

1 Stand with your feet a little wider than shoulder width apart and toes turned out slightly. Keep your upper body upright and relaxed and place your hands on your hips.

2 Tighten both your abdominal and buttock muscles, then bend your knees in line with your toes for 2 counts. Hold the position for 2 counts, then push up through your heels to the starting position for 4 counts.

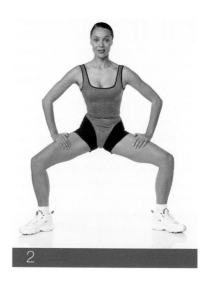

make sure your buttocks remain tight throughout; do not lock your knees

104

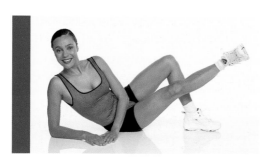

◀ inner thigh raise

Lie on your side with one thigh on top of the other and go up on to your elbow. Bend your top leg and bring it behind the bottom one. Keeping your hips forward, tighten your abdominals and raise the lower leg off the floor for 2 counts, then lower for 2 counts. Build up to 15 to 20 repetitions. Repeat with the other leg.

▶ straight-legged outer thigh raise

Lie on your side with your legs straight, keeping your thighs together and hips facing forwards. Rest your head on your hand. Keeping your hips forward, tighten your abdominal and buttock muscles and raise the top leg for 4 counts, then lower for 4 counts. Repeat on the other side.

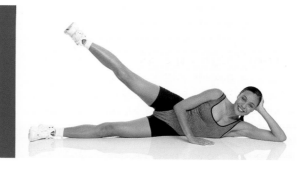

raise your leg from the hip; your toes, knees and hips should all face forwards

bum stretches

▸ outer thigh stretch

Sit with both feet out in front of you. Bend your left leg and cross it over the right to rest outside your right knee. Pull your abdominals in. Now bring your right arm over your left knee and either place your hand on the floor or gently press your left knee in towards your body. Hold the stretch for 15 seconds. Repeat on the other side.

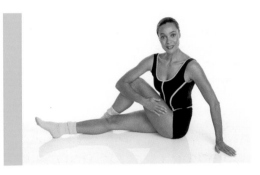

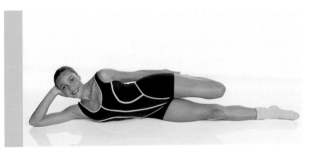

◂ inner thigh stretch

Sit with your back straight, then bend your knees and bring the soles of your feet together. Gently press your knees down towards the floor. Hold this position for 15 seconds.

only press your knees as far as is comfortable to increase the stretch; bring your heels closer to your groin

▸ front thigh stretch

Lie on your side with your legs straight but soft at the knee. Bend the top leg so that your heel is towards your buttocks. Bring your top hand towards your heel and gently bring the heel closer to your buttocks, tilting your pelvis as you do so. Hold for 15 seconds. Repeat on the other side.

make sure your thighs are parallel; do not strain your knee by pulling too hard

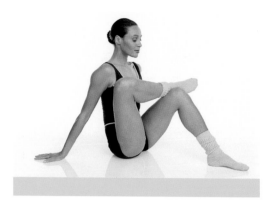

◀ buttock stretch

Sit with one leg straight and the other bent. Cross the bent leg over the knee of the straight leg. Bring the ankle across the knee. Bend the straight leg, placing the foot flat on the floor, and bring the heel towards your buttocks. Place your hands just behind you on the floor for support. Hold for 15 seconds. Repeat with the other leg.

▶ hamstring stretch

From the buttock stretch position, uncross your legs and extend one of them. Bend the other one and let your knee fall to the side, so that the foot faces the inner thigh of the straight leg. Turn your body so that you are in line with the straight leg and place your hands on the floor on either side of it. Tighten your abdominals, then gently ease forward until you feel a stretch on your hamstring, at the back of the thigh. Hold for 15 seconds. Repeat with the other leg.

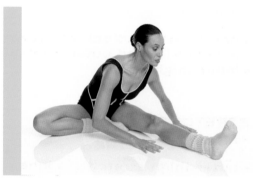

make sure your back is not arched; check that you are leaning forward from your hips; do not bounce or jerk

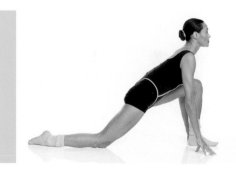

◀ hip flexor stretch

Kneel on one knee with your other leg bent and the foot flat on the floor. You can use a cushion, mat or towel for extra padding. Place your hands on either side of your foot for support. Move your hips forward until you feel a stretch in the front of your left hip. Hold for 15 seconds. Repeat on the other side.

intermediate
bum workout

WARM UP

As for the beginner's workout.

TONING

Spend about 30 seconds on each exercise (or each side, where these are worked separately).

- **one-legged buttock squeeze**
- **straight-legged outer thigh raise**
- **inner thigh raise**
- **wide squat**

107

STRETCHES

Hold each stretch for 15 seconds.

- **outer thigh stretch**
- **front thigh stretch**
- **hamstring stretch**
- **inner thigh stretch**
- **buttock stretch**
- **hip flexor stretch**

If you do not have time to do 2 sets of the toning exercises, do 1 set but perform the movements very slowly, putting your mind to your muscle to create resistance. Or you could do the first two exercises in the morning and the second two in the afternoon.

advanced

work
out

advanced

When you are comfortable with all the exercises in Chapter 9 you can move on to those presented in this section, which are a combination of **advances and variations** on the exercises in the earlier chapters. For the bum exercises, once you have mastered the movements as given here you can progress by using **ankle weights or dynabands** (resistance bands), or even the equipment in the gym! But once again, remember: don't run before

workout

you can walk, and only progress further when the exercises no longer challenge you. By now you will also be very familiar with how to perform abdominal exercises. This is the time really to use your powers of **concentration and visualisation** for quality movement. Be very much aware of how you feel as you perform each exercise. As always, remember to keep your spine in a neutral position and to use slow, controlled movements throughout.

tum exercises

▶ full-length tummy tightener

1 Kneel on all fours, then go down on to your elbows and straighten your right leg, curling the toes under on the floor.

2 Now straighten your left leg, keeping both feet together. Pull your abdominals in tight and lower your hips until your body is a straight line. Hold for 15 to 30 seconds, building up to 1 minute. If you feel strain in your back, either widen your stance or use the position in the intermediate workout.

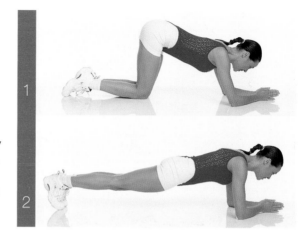

keep your head in line with your body; your back should be completely flat; do not hold your breath

▶ advanced waist tightener

1 If you have any shoulder problems, check with your doctor before doing this exercise. Lie on your side with your body in a straight line and bend your knees slightly. Place your elbow underneath your shoulder and your other hand in front of you on the floor.

2 Tighten your abdominals and push your hips off the ground. Take your hand off the floor and place it on your side. Keeping your body in a straight line, with a slight bend in the knee, hold for 15 seconds, building up to 30 seconds. Repeat on the other side. If you experience problems with your balance, place your hand back on the floor.

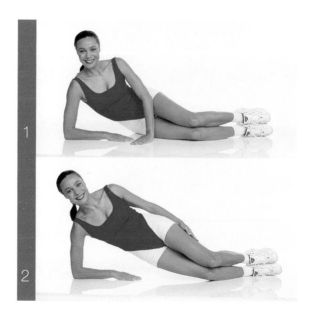

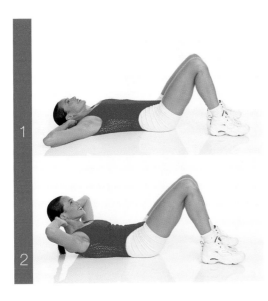

◀ advanced curl-up

1 Lie on your back with your legs bent and feet shoulder width apart. Rest your head on your fingertips with your elbows bent.

2 Tighten your abdominals and curl up to bring your shoulders off the floor for 2 counts, hold for 1 count and then lower for 4 counts. Build up to 15 to 20 repetitions.

do not pull on your head; do not arch your back; keep your elbows back

▶ advanced reverse curl

1 Lie on your back with both knees bent and over your tummy button. Now straighten your legs but keep your knees soft. Place your hands by your sides.

2 Keeping your knees together, tighten your abdominals and tilt your pelvis to curl your buttocks and lower back off the floor. Curl up for 2 counts and slowly roll down for 4 counts. Build up to 15 to 20 repetitions.

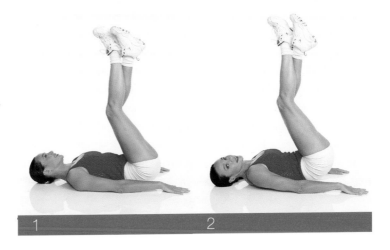

do not rock; do not hold your breath

tum stretches

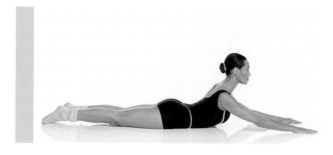

keep your hips still and your feet on the floor; look straight ahead; only come up as far as is comfortable with no strain on your back

▲ abdominal stretch

Lie on your front with your feet together and hips on the floor. Take your hands in front of your head with your arms slightly bent. Push on your hands and lift your head and shoulders off the floor until you feel a stretch in your abdominal muscles. Hold for 15 seconds, building up to 30 seconds.

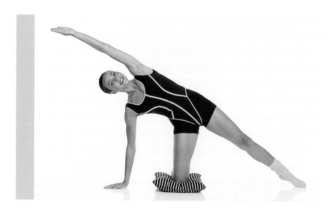

make sure your right knee is directly under your right hip; keep your right hand directly under your right shoulder

▲ side stretch

Kneel on your right knee. Straighten your left leg and take it out directly to the left. Place your right hand flat on the floor on your right side. Bring your left arm over your head to stretch the side of your body. Hold for 15 seconds, building up to 30 seconds. Repeat on the other side.

advanced
tum workout

WARM UP
As for the beginner's workout.

TONING
Spend about 1 minute on the full-length tummy tightener, and about 30 seconds on each of the other exercises (or on each side, where these are worked separately).

- **full-length tummy tightener**
- **advanced waist tightener**
- **advanced curl-up**
- **advanced reverse curl**

STRETCHES
Hold each stretch for 15 to 30 seconds.

- **advanced abdominal stretch** (see page 114)
- **side stretch**   • **full body stretch**

115

You should now be feeling a great sense of achievement as you move closer to your goal of the perfect tum and bum.

Your buttock muscles should now be feeling firmer and much more toned. You can challenge them further with the exercises in this section. Keep your back flat and make every repetition count!

bum exercises

▶ kneeling buttock tightener

1 Kneel on all fours in a 'box' position, with hands and knees on the floor. Now go down on to your elbows, extend your right leg out behind you and bend your knee in line with your hip so that your heel faces the ceiling. Do not raise your foot so high that you arch your back.

2 Squeeze your buttock muscles and raise your right leg for 2 counts, then lower for 2 counts. Build up to 15 or 20 repetitions. Repeat with the other leg.

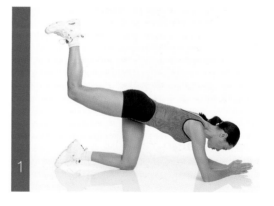
1

keep your hips still and square to the floor and your heel facing the ceiling

▸ lunge

Stand with your feet together in an upright posture. Take a step forward, tighten your abdominal and buttock muscles and bend both knees to 90 degrees. Hold for 1 count, then push up through the front leg to the starting position. Build up to 15 to 20 repetitions. Repeat with the other leg.

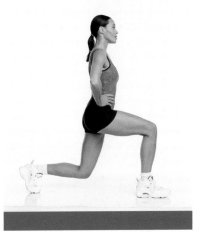

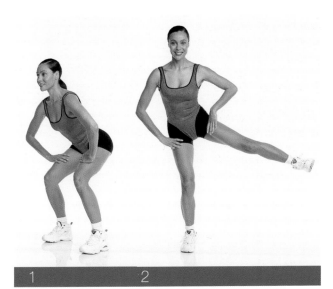

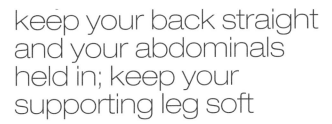

117

◂ squat and side raise

1 Stand with your feet shoulder width apart and toes facing forwards. Place your hands on your hips. Tighten your abdominal and buttock muscles and bend your knees to sit back into your heels in a squat position.

2 With the weight still in your heels, take your right leg out to the side to about 45 degrees. Hold for 1 count, then bring your right leg back in and return to the starting position. Repeat with the left leg. Build up to 15 to 20 repetitions.

keep your back straight and your abdominals held in; keep your supporting leg soft

▸ inner thigh raise

Lie on your side and go up on to your elbows. Bend your top leg and bring your foot to rest on the inner thigh of the bottom leg. Place your hand in front of you for support. Pull your abdominals in. Lift the lower leg for 2 counts, then lower for 2 counts. Build up to 15 to 20 repetitions. Repeat on the other side.

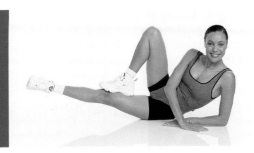

bum stretches

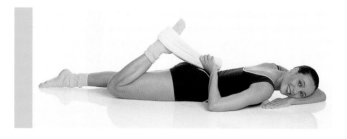

to increase the stretch, lift the knee off the floor slightly; you can hook a towel around your foot

▲ front thigh stretch

Lie on your tummy. Bend your right leg to bring your right heel towards your buttocks. Reach for the heel and gently pull it in until you get a stretch along the front of your thigh. Hold for 15 seconds. Repeat with the other leg.

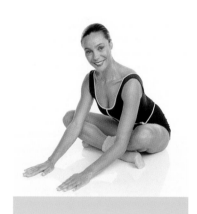

◀ sitting buttock stretch

In a sitting position, cross your legs with the left leg under and right leg over. Place your hands on the floor in front of you. Slowly start walking forwards with your hands until you begin to get a stretch in your right buttock. Hold for 15 seconds. Repeat with your legs crossed the other way.

gently ease forward from the hip; do not hold your breath

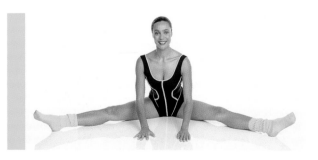

◀ straddle stretch

Sit on the floor with your legs wide apart. Place your hands in front of you on the floor. Bend forwards from the hips and walk your hands forwards until you feel a stretch on the inside and back of your thighs. Hold for 15 seconds.

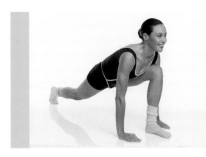

◀ advanced hip flexor stretch
Kneel on your right knee and bend your left knee, placing your left foot on the floor. Place your hands on the floor for support. Now raise your right knee off the ground and straighten your right leg. Lower your hips towards the floor. Hold for 15 seconds. Repeat with the other leg. You should feel the stretch in front of your right hip and in your left buttock. Do not bounce. If you cannot keep the back leg straight let the knee rest on the floor.

advanced
bum workout

119

WARM UP
As for the beginner's workout.

TONING
Spend about 30 seconds on each exercise (or each side, where these are worked separately).

- **kneeling buttock tightener**
- **squat and side raise**
- **lunge**
- **inner thigh raise**

STRETCHES
Hold each stretch for 15 seconds.

- **front thigh stretch**
- **straddle stretch**
- **sitting buttock stretch**
- **advanced hip flexor stretch**

If you are short of time, stick to 1 set of the toning exercises but use ankle weights or dynabands.

the way

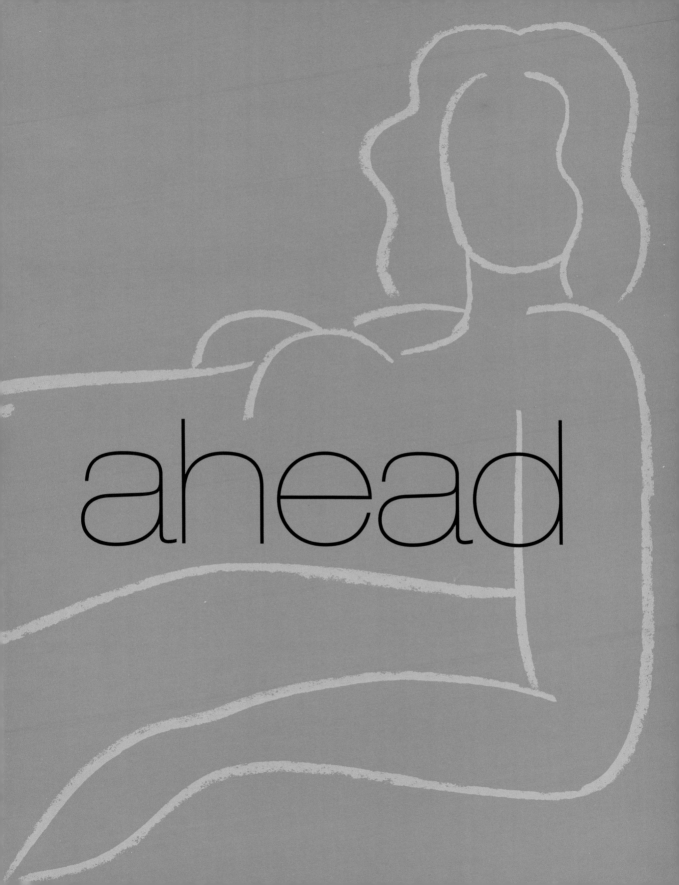

ahead

The following programme of exercise and visualisation is designed to ensure that you maximise your mental and physical energies at each stage of the workout and build up gradually to your goal.

10-minute
tone-up programme

P = posture workout   T = tum workout   B = bum workout

perfect posture: FOUNDATION WORK

M	T	W	T	F	S	S
P	tape	P	tape	P	tape	tape
P	tape	P	tape	P	tape	tape
P	tape	P	tape	P	tape	tape
P	tape	P	tape	P	tape	tape

Do posture exercises 3 times a week and play back your visualisation tape on the other 4 days. After 1 month, you should be ready for the beginner's workout.

BEGINNER'S WORKOUT

M	T	W	T	F	S	S
T	B	tape	T	B	tape	P
T	B	tape	T	B	tape	P
T	B	tape	T	B	tape	P
T	B	tape	T	B	tape	P

Do 3 sessions per week for your tum and bum, divided into 2 toning sessions and 1 for posture. Play your tape on 2 days. After 1 month you should be ready for the intermediate workout.

INTERMEDIATE WORKOUT

M	T	W	T	F	S	S
T	B	T	B	tape	P	rest
T	B	T	B	tape	P	rest
T	B	T	B	tape	P	rest
T	B	T	B	tape	P	rest

As for the beginner's workout, do 3 sessions per week for your tum and bum, divided into 2 toning sessions and 1 for posture. Play your tape on 1 day a week as a reminder and to keep that image of a perfect tum and bum firmly in your mind. After 1 month you should be ready for the advanced workout.

ADVANCED WORKOUT

M	T	W	T	F	S	S
T	B	rest	B	T	P	rest
T	B	tape	B	T	P	rest
T	B	rest	B	T	P	rest
T	B	rest	B	T	P	tape

As before, do 3 sessions per week for your tum and bum, divided into 2 toning sessions and 1 for posture. Play your tape occasionally. You should now have a firm image in your mind that you can call on any time you like to lead you towards your goal. You are much closer to your goal of the perfect tum and bum. Your posture will have improved, as will the general tone of your tum and bum. Don't forget to include aerobic work for a leaner shape, and of course remember to eat healthily.

Well done! You have now completed the full 10-minute tone-up programme. Your posture will have improved and so will your muscle tone. You may now feel ready for a further challenge.

where now?

When you first start to exercise you begin to feel and see improvements fairly quickly, but after a period of time the body tends to plateau and needs to be challenged again.

You can progress further in all sorts of ways. You could apply further resistance to your muscles by investing in a home gym kit. This would include ankle weights, dumbells, dynabands and various different gadgets for your abdominals. You could join a local gym and use the equipment there. You may also want to allow yourself longer to exercise. But if you are still limited to 10 minutes there is another answer – simply split your workout.

For 10-minute tone-ups, splitting your routine means you still exercise for 10 minutes but increase the number of days on which you work out, or the number of times per day you work out – for example, one session in the morning and one in the afternoon or evening. You also increase the intensity of your workout by adding on another set.

The chart on the opposite page sets out a simple routine that you can follow. Aim to build up to two sets of 15 to 20 repetitions.

MONDAY
Morning
- Kneeling buttock tightener 2 sets
- Lunge 2 sets
- Stretch

Evening
- Abdominals 1 set
- Stretch

TUESDAY
- Outer thigh raise 2 sets
- Inner thigh raise 2 sets
- Stretch

WEDNESDAY
- Abdominals 1 set
- Stretch

THURSDAY
- One-legged buttock squeeze 2 sets
- Wide squat 2 sets
- Stretch

FRIDAY
Morning
- Outer thigh raise 2 sets
- Inner thigh raise 2 sets
- Stretch

Evening
- Abdominals 1 set
- Stretch

SATURDAY, SUNDAY
- Free

For the abdominals, I recommend that you stick to 1 set but increase the intensity by varying the speed at which you work out – for example, increasing the number of counts for which you hold or release a contraction – and perhaps add in an extra day.

Once you have achieved your perfect tum and bum you will need to maintain it. This requires less fewer and shorter sessions, reducing your workload to once or twice a week for each muscle group – but when you do exercise you need to make sure you keep up the intensity.

I hope this book will prove a useful resource to help you achieve your goal of a flatter, stronger, more toned tum and bum. It will take a little time, a little effort and lots of consistency – but I know you will do it. Good luck.

index

bibliography

Athletic Ability and the Anatomy of Motion; Rolf Wirhed; Mosby, 1997.

Personal Trainer Manual; Richard Cotton (editor); American Council on Exercise, 1999.

Exercise Physiology; William McArdle, Frank Katch and Victor Katch; Lippincott Williams and Wilkins, 1996.

Abdominal Training; Christopher Norris; A&C Black, 1997.

acknowledgements

In writing a book that involves anatomy and physiology, it is wise to make sure that all the information gathered is up to date and in line with present thinking. I am most grateful to Jane Groffski, BSc Hons Exercise Physiology, BpnEd MAR LicAc, for advice on anatomy and physiology, and to Joy Walters, MSc, Grad Dip Phys (NZ), NCSP, SRP, MACP, chartered physiotherapist, for her advice on posture for tums and bums.

I would also like to express my gratitude to the International Training Seminar and The Atkinson Ball College of Hypnotherapy for skills taught in NLP and Hypnotherapy. My thanks to Laura Washburn for giving me the opportunity to write this book, and to the photographic team for the pictures.

Thanks also to the Leotard Company of The Thatch, Great Billing Park, Northampton NN3 9BL (tel: 01604 416000; fax: 01604 406901) for the lovely outfits.

Lastly, my gratitude as ever to Jamie, my son, for his support and to Greg, my partner, for his encouragement.